PROGRESS IN RADIOPHARMACOLOGY 3

DEVELOPMENTS IN NUCLEAR MEDICINE

VOLUME 2

Other titles in this series

1. Cox, P.H. (ed.): Cholescintigraphy. 1981.
   ISBN 90-247-2524-0

PROGRESS IN RADIOPHARMACOLOGY 3
Selected Topics

Proceedings of the Third European Symposium on Radiopharmacology
held at Noordwijkerhout, The Netherlands, April 22-24, 1982

edited by

PETER H. COX

Head Department of Nuclear Medicine
Rotterdamsch Radio-Therapeutisch Instituut

Co-ordinating Chairman Joint Committee on Radiopharmaceuticals of the
Society of Nuclear Medicine and the European Nuclear Medicine Society

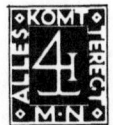

1982

MARTINUS NIJHOFF PUBLISHERS
THE HAGUE / BOSTON / LONDON

Distributors:

for the United States and Canada

Kluwer Boston, Inc.
190 Old Derby Street
Hingham, MA 02043
USA

for all other countries

Kluwer Academic Publishers Group
Distribution Center
P.O. Box 322
3300 AH Dordrecht
The Netherlands

Library of Congress Cataloging in Publication Data   CIP

European Symposium on Radiopharmacology (3rd : 1982 :
   Noordwijkerhout, Netherlands)
   Proceedings of the Third European Symposium on
Radiopharmacology held at Noordwijkerhout, the
Netherlands, April 22-24, 1982.

   (Developments in nuclear medicine ; v. 2)
(Progress in radiopharmacology ; 3)
   Includes index.
   1. Radiopharmaceuticals--Congresses.
2. Radiopharmaceuticals--Metabolism--Congresses.
3. Radioisotopes in pharmacolcgy--Congresses.
I. Cox, Peter H. II. Title. III. Title: Proceedings
of the 3rd European Symposium on Radiopharmacology
held at Noordwijkerhout, the Netherlands, April
22-24, 1982. IV. Series. V. Series: Progress in
radiopharmacology ; 3. [DNLM: 1. Radioisotopes--
Diagnostic use--Congresses. W1 DE998KF v.2 / WN 445
E89 1982]
RM852.E97 1982   616.07'575   82-18823
ISBN   978-94-009-7671-9

ISBN 978-94-009-7671-9   ISBN 978-94-009-7669-6 (eBook)
DOI 10.1007/978-94-009-7669-6

CONTENTS

PREFACE

The publication of this volume, which is based upon presentations made to the Third European Symposium on Radiopharmacology at Noordwijkerhout, April 22 - 24, 1982, is indicative of the continued interest in this sub-branch of Nuclear Medicine. The transactions of the first two meetings were published as Progress in Radiopharmacology, Volumes 1 and 2 by Elsevier/North-Holland Biomedical Press. We are particularly pleased to have reached an agreement with Martinus Nijhoff Publishers to include Progress in Radiopharmacology 3 in the series Developments in Nuclear Medicine. This not only ensures the continuity of the series but by including it in a series of Nuclear Medical Monographs the availability of the text to more general readers, for background information, is greatly enhanced.

As with the previous two volumes each of the three topics has been so treated as to relate the biodistribution of the radiopharmaceuticals to normal and pathophysiological conditions to provide background information for the practising nuclear medical specialist. Special attention has been given to European activities but these have been clearly placed in context in relation to developments from outside Europe.

The Third European Symposium on Radiopharmacology was held under the auspices of the European Joint Commitee on Radiopharmaceuticals of the European Nuclear Medicine Society and the Society of Nuclear Medicine Europe. Solco Nuclear, Basle, provided both financial and material support and I would like to thank Dr M. de Schrijver, Mr. I. Waser and Mrs. E. Rüfenacht for their continued help and encouragement.

My secretary Mrs. M. Busker co-ordinated the correspondence and prepared the camera-ready manuscript in its final form. This is the fourth camera-ready book which she has prepared during the last three years on top of her normal duties. I can only admire her enthusiasm and energy. Colleagues from 14 countries participated in the meeting and from their deliberations this volume has emerged to provide, we hope, a useful source of basic information.

Peter H. Cox
Rotterdam.

CONTRIBUTORS

Aprile, C.
— Fondazione Clinica del Lavoro, Istituto di Medicina del Lavoro, Università di Pavia, Servizio di Medicina Nucleare, Pavia, Italy

Bazin, J.P.
— Unité de Radiobiologie Clinique (U66, INSERM) Villejuif, France

Britton, J.
— Department of Nuclear Medicine, St. Bartholomew's Hospital, London, U.K.

Cox, P.H.
— Department of Nuclear Medicine, Rotterdamsch Radio-Therapeutisch Instituut, Rotterdam, The Netherlands

Frühling, J.
— Laboratoire des Radio-Isotopes, Service de Radio-thérapie, Institut J. Bordet, Université Libre de Bruxelles, Belgium

Füger G.F.
— Division of Nuclear Medicine, Department of Radiology and Central Roentgen Institute, Carl Franzens University, Graz, Austria

Jonckheer, M.H.
— Department of Radioisotopes and Division of Vascular Surgery, Academisch Ziekenhuis, Vrije Universiteit, Brussels, Belgium

Kloster, G.
— Institut für Chemie 1 (Nuklearchemie), KFA Jülich, FRG

Leeuw de, P.W.
— Department of Medicine, Zuiderziekenhuis, Rotterdam, The Netherlands

Limouris, G.
— Department of Nuclear Medicine, Hygeias Melathron Hospital of the National Bank Greece, Athens, Greece

Marcuse, H.R.
— Netherlands Cancer Institute, Antoni van Leeuwen-hoekhuis, Amsterdam, The Netherlands

Ott, E.
— Division of Nuclear Medicine, Department of Radiology and Central Roentgen Institute, Carl Franzens University, Graz, Austria

Pfeiffer, G.
— Swiss Federal Institute for Reactor Research, Würenlingen (EIR), Switzerland

Rhodes, C.G.
— MRC Cyclotron Unit, Hammersmith Hospital, London, U.K.

Shukla, S.K.
— Istituto di Chimica Nucleare, Rome, Italy

Tennvall, J.
— Department of Oncology, University Hospital, Lund, Sweden

Tyrrell, D.A.
— Amersham International plc, Buckinghamshire, U.K.

Verbruggen, A.
— Laboratory of Radiopharmacy, University of Leuven, Academic Hospital St. Rafaël, Leuven, Belgium

White, Th.   - Department of Clinical Physiology, University
                        Lund, Sweden

Wiebe, L.I.   - University of Alberta and Cross Cancer Instit
                        Edmonton, Canada

Zolle, I.   - Department of Nuclear Medicine, Second Medica
                        Clinic, University of Vienna, Austria

INTRODUCTION

The Third European Symposium on Radiopharmacology was held at Noordwijker-hout, The Netherlands, from 22 - 24 April 1982. Representations from 14 countries participated in the meeting emphasizing the continued interest in this type of specialized symposia. In the tradition of the first two meetings three selected topics: Brain, Kidney and Endocrinology were dealt with in depth by invited speakers together with original work submitted in poster form. At the request of a number of participants a free paper session was also held for the first time and also a half day meeting for technicians under the auspices of the VANG (the Dutch Society for Nuclear Medical Technicians).

In the main meeting the session on renal diseases provided some interesting original data concerning the evaluation of renal circulation using Xenon which was complemented by reviews of the reagents available to study glomerular and tubule function. A comparison of biodistribution data on reagents for scinti-graphy led to the conclusion that although Tc DMSA shows the highest degree of concentration in the renal cortex the characteristics of Tc glucoheptonate give a better visualization of the organ. A new reagent Aprotinin was introduced which shows a high affinity for the renal cortex, no liver or spleen uptake and an extremely low urinary excretion. These characteristics may prove to be of great value both in evaluating relative renal function and in the detection of space occupying lesions.

The presentations on Brain clearly demonstrated the value of positron emission studies for the elucidation of function and it is unfortunate that such techniques will be limited to a few specialist centres. The criteria for the use of Tc^{99m} DMSA labelling kits for cisternography aroused much discussion partic-ularly with regard to the pyrogen testing of "in house" preparations. It was clearly emphasized that only eluates from new generators should be used in order to minimize the risk factor and also that the formulation was extremely important to prevent toxic reactions. Against this background In^{111} DTPA showed up as a reliable reagent with minimal risks.

The section on Endocrinology brought a variety of papers on new approaches ranging from Thallium uptake in thyroid carcinoma, Iodine-131 dosimetry in therapy and the effect of generators on Technetium uptake in the thyroid to new pancreas reagents and estrogens as potential agents for the detection of prostate carcinoma.

Clearly many problems remain to be solved and from these discussions a number of research topics could be initiated.

Each section of this book presents the "state of the art", in a European setting, to provide useful background information for practising nuclear medi specialists and other disciplines.

P.H. Cox

Rotterdam, June 1982.

KIDNEY

THE KIDNEY: PATHOPHYSIOLOGY

K. BRITTON

INTRODUCTION

While it is not known quite how the kidneys work, it is clear what they do.
They maintain the internal environment: salt and water balance, acid and osmolal
control; and the levels of potassium, calcium and phosphate ions. Metabolites
such as urea, uric acid, creatinine and sulphate are not retained whilst
important substrates such as amino acids, bicarbonate and glucose are conserved.
The active derivative of vitamin D, erythropoietin, and the enzyme Renin are
secreted into the blood.

The organization of the kidney depends on combinations and juxtapositions
of tubes and loops of living cells and a hierarchy of control systems. These
are at a cellular level, at a loop level, at the level of the two populations
of nephrons, at the whole kidney level and at the circulatory level with humor-
al and autonomic interactions. Using radionuclides only a small proportion of
these functions and control systems are susceptible to study at present. But two
very important functions can be determined: uptake function, the ability of the
kidney to take up substances from the blood, and parenchymal: transit function,
an index of salt and water reabsorption.

An understanding of renal pathophysiology is necessary for the intelligent
use of renal radiopharmaceuticals and conversely a knowledge of the renal handling of radiopharmaceuticals is necessary to the understanding of disorder of
renal function in an individual patient. An appreciation is required of the
intact nephron hypothesis, the importance of tubulo-glomerular balance, the
different properties of the two populations of nephrons and the mechanism of
cortical nephron autoregulation.

The renal handling of some radiopharmaceuticals

Radioiodinated orthoiodohippurate, I-OIH, when introduced into the blood
equilibrates with extracellular fluid and with red cells. I-OIH is weakly protein

bound to the extent of 70%. This weak protein binding reduces the glomerular
filtration of I-OIH from a potential 20% of the renal blood supply to about 6
((100-70)% of 20%) but the protein binding is insufficient to prevent the
avid uptake and active transport of I-OIH into the cells of the proximal tubu
and into their tubular lumens. The uptake and secretion of I-OIH takes place
the proximal tubules of both cortical and juxtamedullary nephrons. The millig
amounts used in radionuclide studies is not rate limiting. The uptake is rela
to the blood supply rate to the proximal tubes. Even in acute tubular necrosi
active transport of I-OIH continues into the proximal tubular cell, unlike [99]
labelled gluconate. However in acute tubular necrosis and other causes of acu
tubular dysfunction, such as some forms of the nephrotic syndrome and acute
glomerulo-nephritis, the active transport of I-OIH out of the tubular cell in
the lumen is inhibited. This causes a prolongation of the residence time of
I-OIH in the proximal tubular cell and is refered to as "parenchymal stasis".

Competition with the active transport carrier mechanism by other compoun
is recognized. The obvious competitor is para-amino hippurate, PAH, when infu
sions of PAH in gram quantities for the classical clearance techniques were
compared with simultaneous I-OIH infusions in milligram amounts. This is the
main reason for the apparently lower clearance of I-OIH than PAH in such stud
(1). Drugs of the penicillin series and probenecid are competitors. Some
contrast media for intravenous urography, IVU, appear to contain a small percentage of some tubular secreted impurity and I-OIH studies are not recommend
within 8 hours of an IVU.

[51]Cr EDTA (ethylene diamine tetracetate) and [99]Tc[m] DTPA (diethylene tria
mine pentacetate), using kits from certain manufacturers (2) show virtually n
protein binding and are glomerular filtered. However radioiodinated iothalama
and diatrizoate have variable protein binding up to 10% in man and correction
for this in plasma samples, for example, by charcoal extraction of the free
component may be necessary to prevent underestimation of the GFR.

[99]Tc[m] DMSA is, like the older mercury labelled compounds, taken up and
fixed in the cells of the proximal tubules (3). It would be ideal if this
compound was only fixed to renal parenchyme and not excreted in the urine, bu
the latter occurs if there is oxidation during preparation, or before use. Th
stability of the preparation depends on the particular kit used. The clinical
requirements for the use of DMSA include the identification of parenchymal sc
infarcts or regional ischaemia and small space occupying lesions as defects i
uptake. Positive uptake indicates the normality of renal tissues in the uro-

graphic "pseudo-tumour" and the presence of renal tissue remnants when the kidney is not evident urographically.

A tubular secreted $^{99}Tc^m$ labelled rival to I-OIH such as $^{99}Tc^m$ DADS (4) is being actively sought but no definitive successor has been established yet.

Physiological models

The crucial requirement for understanding kidney function using radio-pharmaceuticals is the creation of a physiological model that is the best compromise of the realistic and simplistic. This is called an isomorphic model. The second requirement is to recognize that the validity of the isomorphic model is the only justification for a particular method of analysis if its results are going to be used to assess renal function. A compartment model must be valid for compartmental analysis to be valid. A linear model must be valid for deconvolution analysis to be valid. The loss of substances from the blood and extracellular fluid spaces to the kidney is most isomorphically modelled using a compartmental model and the movement of substances from their point of uptake along the million nephrons is most isomorphically modelled using the linear system approach, to give the tracers transit time. Conversely a compartmental model is not an isomorphic or valid way of representing a kidney made up of a million tubes. A fundamental assumption of a compartmental model is that the rate of mixing within a compartment is rapid compared to the rate of exchange between compartments. Thus it is not true both on theoretical grounds (5) and empirically (6) that the components derived from the exponential analysis of the xenon washout curve represent flows to different parts of the kidney.

A compartment model with exponential analysis is used for the clearance of tracers from the blood or plasma to the kidney to estimate the uptake function of the kidney, whether this be the effective renal plasma flow or glomerular filtration rate depends on the compound used. It should be noted that the definition of renal "clearance" has changed from movement of a substance from blood to urine to movement of a substance from blood to kidney.

The intact nephron hypothesis

Bricker (7) proposed that "surviving nephrons of the diseased kidney largely retain their essential functional integrity". Thus whether a tubule is damaged or a glomerulus is damaged, the hypothesis implies that the whole nephron fails to function. For this to be so, the Glomural Filtration Rate, GFR, the Renal Plasma Flow, RPF, and tubular uptake and secretion must be indissolubably inter-related. If this is true then the filtration fraction (GFR/RPF) of one kidney is equal to that of the other. This may be confirmed experimentally (1). Thus if one sets out the problem "what is the GFR of the left kidney"? in table I, then the answer 20 ml/min is self evident.

Table I. Intact nephron hypothesis

	left kidney	right kidney	left % total
GFR ml/min	?	80	?
ERPF ml/min	100	400	20%
Filtration function	?	0.2	

This result in turn implies that the percentage contribution of one kidney to total function is the same whether a glomerular filtered agent or a tubular secreted or tubularly fixed agent is used. That this is generally true has been confirmed many times using pairs of the following: ^{131}I-OIH, ^{99}Tc^{m} DTPA, ^{197}Hg chlormedrin, ^{99}Tc^{m} DMSA. Finally the hypothesis implies that functioning nephrons are working in a similar way whichever kidney they are in. This may be demonstrated by the fact that the peaks of a pair of normal renograms occur at the same time; by the fact that a kidney with half the normal number of nephro e.g. due to pyelonephritis, has a peak to its kidney curve at the same time as that of the contralateral normal kidney (in the absence of renovascular dis-order) although of course the amplitude of the kidney curve is less; and by th similarity of intrarenal flow distribution in the left and right kidney in essential hypertension (8). It may be noted that situations may be made to occur where the intact nephron hypothesis does not hold in order to investigat the control mechanisms, as shown by unsteady state conditions and by experimen al alterations of the intrerenal flow distribution of one kidney only. The mechanisms on which the intact nephron hypothesis is based include tubulo-glomerular balance and autoregulation.

Tubulo-glomerular balance

This term is used to describe the interrelationship between tubular re-absorption and glomerular filtration. The more salt that is filtered the more salt is reabsorbed in proportion.

The proximal tubular reabsorption of salt and water occurs in two main

ways: by active transport through the cell, possibly controlled by a "natri-
uretic hormone", and by passive movement through the "tight" junctions and
along the intercellular space. Fromter (9) demonstrated in the rat kidney that
up to 60% of filtered salt and water could be reabsorbed passively. In the
human a smaller percentage of the filtered salt and water reabsorbed by the
tubule depends on passive forces. Earley and Friedler (10) demonstrated the
importance of peritubular capillary pressure in the control of salt and water
reabsorption and the many studies in this field (11) demonstrate that a fall in
peritubular capillary pressure relative to intratubular pressure enhances salt
and water reabsorption (as occurs in renovascular disorder) and that a rise in
intratubular pressure relative to peritubular capillary pressure similarly
enhances salt and water reabsorption (as occurs with resistance to outflow).
One consequence of both situations is that the rate of tubular movement of a
non reabsorbable solute is slower than before and thus the renal parenchymal
transit time of such a solute is prolonged. Therefore prolongation of the radio-
actively labelled non reabsorbable tracers I-OIH and $^{99}Tc^m$ DTPA parenchymal
transit times is a clear indication of a raised intrarenal and pelvic pressure
consequent on the presence of significant outflow obstruction. Such prolongation
of nephron transit time in the presence of outflow obstruction is well established in stop flow studies in animals where lissamine green was used as the non
reabsorbable solute (12). In this way the problem of the diagnosis of outflow
obstruction is transduced into that of measuring parenchymal transit time (13).

The cortical and juxtamedullary nephrons
The kidney contains two populations of nephrons. The cortical nephrons
mainly conserve salt, glucose and amino acids and have the property of autoregulation, that is the ability to maintain a constant renal blood-flow and
glomerular filtration rate in the face of psyiological changes in blood-
pressure. The juxtamedullary nephrons mainly conserve water and their blood-
flow is directly related to the prevailing blood-pressure. The properties of
the two populations are summarized in table II.

Cortical nephron autoregulation.
This depends on the renin containing juxtaglomerular apparatus, JGA. A
rise in blood-pressure causes a rise in afferent arteriolar flow, a rise in GFR,
so more salt is filtered and more is delivered to the distal tubule, so more is
absorbed at the JGA. In response to this more renin is released locally in the

Table II. Features of cortical and juxtamedullary nephrons

	cortical nephrons	juxtamedullary nephrons
Percentage of all nephrons	85%	15%
Afferent arteriole	thick and muscular	thin
Efferent arteriole	thin	thick and muscular
Juxtaglomerular apparatus	present	not present
Local renin angiotensin system	present	not present
Effect of a rise in B/P	autoregulation	increased flow
Effect of a fall in B/P	autoregulation	decreased flow
Loops of Henle	short	long

JGA, more angiotensin I is produced locally and converted into angiotensin I
the Angiotensin Converting Enzyme, ACE, locally. Angiotensin II increases
afferent arteriolar tone and thus afferent arteriolar flow is returned to nc
and GFR returns to normal. The response takes about 45 sec. In this way each
cortical nephron is adjusted appropriately to any physiological circulatory
change. Conversely a fall in blood-pressure leads to a fall of GRF, a reduce
filtration of salt and reduced delivery of salt to the JGA so that there is
fall of the local JGA angiotensin formation and a relaxation of afferent art
lar tone. The renin is ejected into the systemic circulation where it leads
an increase in circulation angiotensin II and consequent peripheral vascocon
struction and aldosterone release. The latter situation is mimicked by renovascular disorder of large or small renal arteries so that discharge of reni
into the renal vein is elevated and because of the reduction of peritubular
capillary pressure, the parenchymal transit time of I-OIH or $^{99}Tc^{m}$ DTPA is p
longed giving rise to the delayed peak of the renogram in functionally signi
ant renovascular disorder. If however there is a pathological fall in blood-
pressure or volume, then artrial stretch receptors become activated and incr
ed sympathetic discharge overrides renal autoregulation and causes afferent
arteriolar constriction, a decrease in glomerular filtration rate, a decreas

peritubular capillary pressure and compensatory salt and water reabsorption. The sympathetic discharge also constricts the efferent arterioles of juxta-medullary nephrons causing a further fall in medullary blood-flow enhancing the osmolal gradient and water conservation. Oliguria is the consequence and the grossly prolonged parenchymal transit time gives a pair of symmetrical continuously rising kidney curves to a plateau with I-OIH or $^{99}Tc^m$ DTPA. What is initially a natural response to a fall in blood-pressure or volume may thus progress to incipient acute renal failure. It may be noted that in some renal disorders, the requirements of the control systems of the kidney override those of the body, e.g. renovascular hypertension, whereas in other conditions the requirements of the body override the control systems of the kidney, e.g. acute renal failure.

Clinical problems

In essential hypertension the function of the two kidneys is equal. It has been known that the effective renal plasma flow is reduced below normal. It is now being shown that this is due to a reduction in the flow to the cortical nephrons to around 75% of total as compared with the normal 85% whereas that to the juxtamedullary nephrons remains normal (8). It has been postulated that the genetic defect in the kidney in essential hypertension may be expressed as an excessive autoregulatory response to normal physiological rises in blood pressure (14). This is supported by the finding that the drug captopril, which is an ACE inhibitor in the production of angiotensin II as in the juxtaglomerular apparatus, increases cortical nephron flow to an even supranormal level, 92% on average.

Renovascular hypertension

This may be defined as being present in those patients in whom an occlusive lesion or lesions of the large or small renal arteries are associated with a particular pattern of renal function and in whom surgical repair or bypass of the lesion or nephrectomy relieves the hypertension. If no surgery is undertaken the diagnosis must remain in doubt although the functional pattern may be typical. The crux of the matter is whether successful surgery to one or both kidneys will cause relief of hypertension. The functional pattern that is currently used is that the renal vein remain activity of the suspected kidney should be over one and a half times that of the "normal" kidney. This does pose problems however because much of the renin leaving the renal vein entered by the renal artery as

renin has a half life of 30 min in the circulation. A kidney with a normal ra
of renin production whose blood-flow is halved will have a twice normal renal
vein renin activity. Thus id ally the rate of renin production which is equal
to (ERPF x Renin(A-V) difference) should be used instead. This is illustrated
in table III where a small kidney with apparent renovascular disorder with a
renal vein renin ratio small to normal of 7 : 4 = 1.75 has no excess renin
production.

Table III. Renal vein renin in renovascular disorder

<table>
<tr><td colspan="2">proximal
inferior vena cava
5 units</td></tr>
<tr><td>small kidney
7 units/ml
ERPF 100 ml/min</td><td>normal kidney
4 units/ml
ERPF 400 ml/min</td></tr>
<tr><td colspan="2">distal
inferior vena cava
3 units</td></tr>
<tr><td colspan="2">renin production = 100 x (7-3) = 400 units/min
renin production = 400 x (4-3) = 400 units/min</td></tr>
</table>

The criteria for established unilateral functionally significant renovas·
cular disorder in a ^{123}I-OIH gamma camera study are: an uptake function of le:
than 43% of total; a mean whole kidney transit time of over 60 sec later than
the normal side or over 270 sec, with a normal pelvic calyceal system and pel\
transit time, this latter excluding outflow disorder.

Renal outflow disorders

These are common and dilatation of the pelvic and/or calyces radiologica]
are common. Loin pain is common and the association of loin pain and a dilated
renal pelvis does not mean that operation on a dilated renal pelvis is indicat
It is only indicated if there is obstruction which means there is an abnormal
resistance to urine flow even although urine flow is maintained. One consequer
of this obstruction is a rise in renal and pelvic pressure with increased salt
and water reabsorption and a prolonged parenchymal transit time. Another consa
quence is reduction of the blood-supply of the non-autoregulating juxtamedulla
nephrons leading to their atrophy so that urinary concentration and hydrogen i

ion secretion are impaired. The resistance to outflow may be tested by inducing
a diuresis, typically with the diuretic frusemide which inhibits active chloride
transport in the thick ascending limb of the loop of Henle. The recommended dose
is 0.3 - 0-5 mg/kg for adults and 1 mg/kg for children, injected 20 min after
the start of the study or later if the pelvis is not visualized. The resultant
diuresis depends on the number of nephrons present. When these are reduced ten-
fold or when renal perfusion is poor with hypotension or hypovolaemia no response
to frusemide may be seen. The resistance to outflow for example at the pelvic
ureteric junction may be overcome by a diuresis particularly when nephron function
is good inspite of there being a higher than normal pressure in the renal and
urinary system. The elasticity of the pelvis will also determine the degree of
resistance to outflow which may be overcome. Thus in states of "mild" obstruction discrepancies are likely to occur between the renal parenchymal transit time
which is related to the intrarenal and urinary system pressure and the resistance
to outflow as assessed by a forced diuresis. This is summarized in table IV. It is
helpful to estimate both indices of outflow disorder in practice.

Table IV. The evaluation of renal outflow disorder

degree of obstruction	intrarenal and pelvic pressure	parenchymal transit time	response to frusemide
none	normal	normal	normal
mild	elevated	prolonged	normal
moderate	elevated	prolonged	impaired
severe	elevated	prolonged	none

Note if renal function is poor there may be no response
    to frusemide in the absence of obstruction

In conclusion, a knowledge of renal pathophysiology is the basis of renal
nuclear medicine which makes a major contribution to the management of patients
with renal disease.

12

REFERENCES

1. Britton KE, Brown NJG In: Clinical Renography, Lloyd-Luke Ltd, London, p. 1-298, 1971.

2. Carlsen JE, Miller ML, Lund JO, Trap-Jensen J, J. nucl. Med. 21:126, 198

3. Arnold RW, Subramanian G, McAfee JG, J. nucl. Med. 16:357, 1975.

4. Klingensmith WG, Gerhold JP, Fritzberg AR, J. nucl. Med. 22:38, 1981.

5. Britton KE, Brown NJG, Bluhm MM, Lancet II: 822, 1971.

6. Slotkoff LM, Logan A, Jose P. D'Avella J, Eisner GM, Circ. Res. 28:158,

7. Bricker NS, Morrin PAF, Kime SW, Amer. J. Med. 28:77, 1960.

8. Gruenewald SM, Nimmon CC, Nawaz MK, Britton KE, Clin. Sci. 61:385, 1981.

9. Fromter E, Rumrich G, Ullrich KJ, Pflugers Arch. 343:189, 1973.

10. Earley LE, Friedler RM, J. clin. Invest. 43:542, 1966.

11. De Wardener HE, Amer. J. Physiol. 235:163, 1978.

12. Rector FC, Bremner FP, Seldin DW, J. clin. Invest. 45:590, 1966.

13. Britton KE, Nimmon CC, Whitfield HN, Hendry WF, Wickham JEA, Lancet I:90 1979.

14. Britton KE, Lancet II:900, 1981.

STUDIES OF THE RENAL CIRCULATION WITH RADIOXENON:
POSSIBILITIES AND LIMITATIONS

P.W. de LEEUW, W.H. BIRKENHÄGER

INTRODUCTION

The kidney is a highly vascularized organ, which receives 20-25% of the
cardiac output. About 80% of its blood-supply passes through the outer cortex,
while the remainder perfuses subcortical and medullary regions. Quantitative
information about the blood-flow to and in the kidney is essential for a good
comprehension of renal function in health and disease. In particular, this
applies to those situations where a reduction in kidney flow causes or perhaps
maintains en elevated blood-pressure.

Several methods have been developed for estimating renal perfusion quantitatively. These include clearance procedures, dye-dilution methods and the inert
as washout technique. In this paper we will focus our attention on the measurement of renal blood-flow by means of ^{133}Xenon-washout.

Theoretical considerations (fig. 1)

The principles of the inert gas washout technique are based on the work by
Kety (1). For any substance carried to an organ in the blood, it is evident that
the amount (Q_a), which is brought in within a time-interval ∇t, must equal the
amount of that substance which during the same time-interval leaves the organ
(Q_v) plus the amount which is accumulated and metabolized in that organ. In the
case of an inert unmetabolizable substance such as radioxenon, no conversion takes
place. Therefore, the total quantity of the substance accumulating in the organ
(Q_i) can be described as:

$$\frac{\Delta Q_i}{\Delta t} = \frac{Q_a}{\Delta t} - \frac{Q_v}{\Delta t} \qquad (1)$$

If it is assumed that flow rates (F) for arterial and venous blood are equal
and constant and if the arterial and venous blood represent the only significant

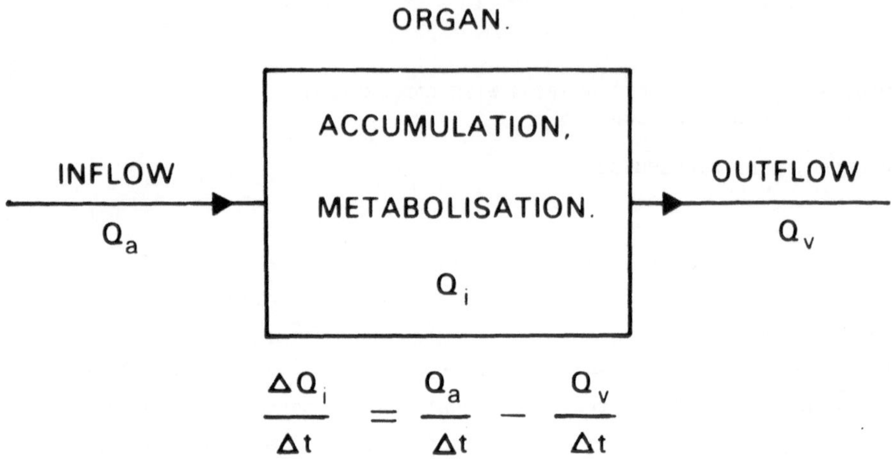

ORGAN.

Fig. 1. Inflow of substance Q in organ equals outflow of that substance plus accumulated and metabolized amount in that organ. For explanation see text.

pathways of entrance and exit for the organ, then equation (1) can be rewritt as:

$$\frac{dQ_i}{dt} = F(C_a - C_v) \qquad (2)$$

where $\frac{dQi}{dt}$ represents the disappearance of tracer per unit of time and C_a and the concentration of the tracer in arterial and venous blood. Immediately aft a bolus injection of xenon into the renal artery, its concentration in arteri. blood falls to zero and therefore:

$$\frac{dQ_i}{dt} = F \times C_v \qquad (3)$$

Even when assuming a rapid equilibration between blood and tissue, concentrat. of xenon in these compartments are not equal because of differences in solubi. The concentration of xenon in tissue (C_i) can be derived from the partition c efficient:

$$\lambda = \frac{C_i}{C_v} \qquad (4)$$

From the combination of (3) and (4) one obtains the formula:

$$\frac{dQ_i}{dt} = \frac{FxC_i}{\lambda} \tag{5}$$

Since $C_i = \frac{Q_i}{V_i}$, where V_i is the total volume of tissue in which the xenon is dissolved, equation (5) can be rearranged to:

$$\frac{dQ_i}{Q_i} = \frac{-Fdt}{V_i x \lambda} \tag{6}$$

The last equation can be integrated to the general form:

$$Q_t = Q_o e - (\frac{F}{V_i x \lambda}) t \tag{7}$$

where Q_t and Q_o represent the amount of xenon (Q_i) at times o and t. When the partition coefficient is known, monitoring the disappearance of xenon from the organ allows calculation of flow per unit volume of tissue or, if the specific gravity is known, per unit mass of tissue.

The equations are valid not only for total organ flow but also for specific regions within an organ. In the case of n parallel open compartments the disappearance curve describes the summation of n different components.

In the heart, a single exponential decay curve can be obtained, but the kidney is characterized by a multiexponential curve. There is still uncertainty, however, about the number of terms needed to describe the washout curve of xenon from the human kidney.

At this point it is necessary to discuss some of the criticisms which have been raised against the xenon washout method as a measure of renal blood-flow. There are a number of assumptions which have not been fully evaluated. First of all, it is assumed that after injection rapid and complete mixing of the indicator occurs in arterial blood, but unfortunately there are no data to substantiate this. Complete mixing may not occur especially at very high flow rates, which in turn may affect the tissue: blood-partition coefficient, another factor which is supposed to be constant. If complete equilibration of the gas between blood and tissue cannot be achieved, then the disappearance constant will be determined both by the diffusional characteristics of the gas as well by the capillary removal rate.

From these purely theoretical considerations one would expect, therefore, that the xenon washout technique becomes more accurate as blood-flow decreases Further prerequisites are that during the time of measurement flow in the compartment under study remains constant, that there is no recirculation of the tracer and that tissue volume remains constant. The latter may not be the case in the kidney during, for instance, saline diuresis or elevated ureteral pressu Thus, since the xenon washout technique measures flow per unit of volume, the disappearance constant will not be altered when significant changes in flow ar accompanied by parallel changes in organ volume. This problem, however, may be circumvented by measuring renal flow simultaneously by another technique such hippuran clearance.

Apart from these theoretical drawbacks, there is the crucial question as which anatomical areas in the kidney define the various components of the wash curve. Thorburn and associates (3) compared the results of ^{85}Kr washout curves autoradiographs in the dog kidney and demonstrated that the most rapid compone (C_1) was analogous to outer cortical flow. Although the authors ascribed the co ponents with longer disappearance time to other areas (outer medulla, inner medulla and perirenal fat), there is no longer any justification for such a distinction (4-6). A great number of studies have been followed since, but uncertainty remains with respect to the physiological meaning of the slow compone of washout curves. Nevertheless the available data seem to indicate that it is reasonable to consider component I flow rate as a measure of total cortical blood-flow. The percentual distribution of the tracer in this compartment in relation to the total amount of radioactivity may be taken as the fraction of total renal flow perfusing the cortex (3-6). However, this does not necessaril imply a distribution over cortical versus juxtamedullary nephrons, since the washout in the latter may be part of the fast-flow component (7).

Although it is clear that the exact meaning of xenon washout curves with respect to the kidney is still open to dispute, a number of interesting result have been obtained with this method, as will be discussed below.

Application in clinical medicine

Since many disease states involving the kidney are characterized by a reduction in renal blood-flow, it is not surprising that a number of investigators have tried to demonstrate a defect in cortical perfusion. Although the cannulation of the renal artery may be cumbersome, the registration of xenon

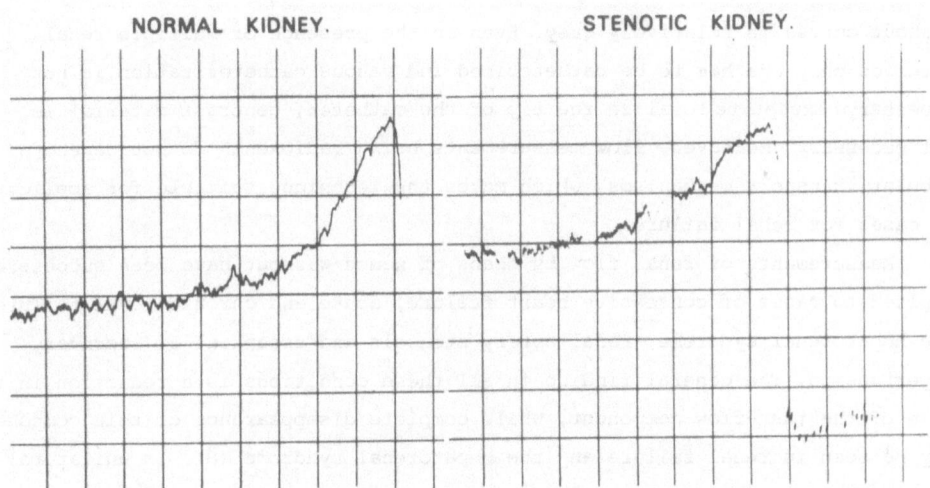

Fig. 2. Comparison of xenon washout curves from a normal (left) and a stenotic (right) kidney. Note slower disappearance of tracer from stenotic kidney.

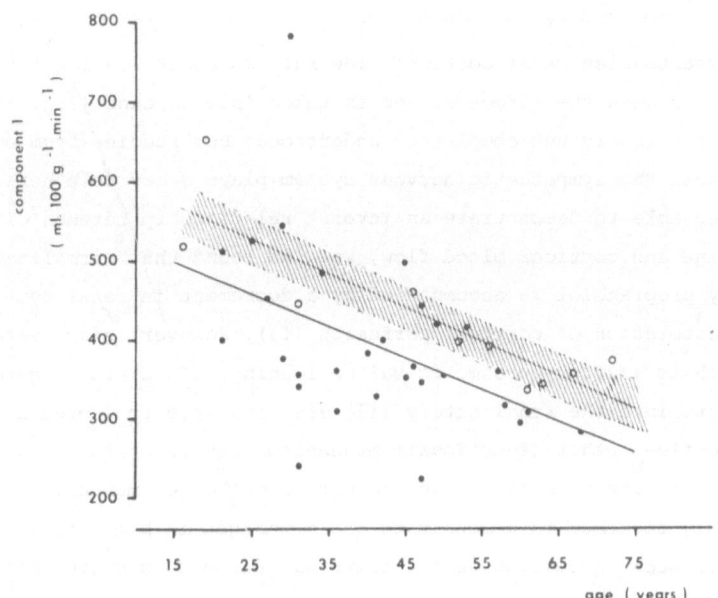

Fig. 3. Relationship between component I flow rate and age in essential hypertension. Dashed area represents 95% confidence interval for normal subjects.

washout curves is relatively easy. Even in the presence of multiple renal
arteries only one has to be catheterized and venous catheterization is not
necessary. Except to localize the tip of the catheter, contrast material is
not necessary. Moreover, flow measurements using radioxenon do not depend on
tubular transport mechanisms, which makes the technique suitable for applicati
to cases for renal failure.

Measurements of renal flow by means of xenon washout have been successful
applied to cases of congestive heart failure, acute and chronic renal failure,
the hepatorenal syndrome, renal artery stenosis and essential or secondary
hypertension. The general finding in all these conditions is a reduction in th
size of the fast-flow component, while complete disappearance of this componen
may be seen in renal failure and the hepatorenal syndrome (8). In unilateral
renal artery stenosis striking differences between the stenotic and the contra
lateral kidney may be found. A significant stenosis results in a decrease in
the rapid component flow rate without redistribution (9). When a washout curve
from a stenotic kidney is compared to one from a normal kidney, a reduction in
component I flow rate in the former seems already evident at first sight
(fig. 2).

In essential hypertension renal cortical flow rate is about 20% lower tha
in normals (10,11) even when the effect of age is taken into account (fig. 3).
The cause of this reduction is not completely understood, but studies from our
laboratory suggest that the sympathetic nervous system plays a key role here.
Not only have we been able to demonstrate an inverse relationship between circulating noradrenaline and cortical blood flow, we also found that normalizati
of blood-pressure by propranolol is accompanied by a decrement in renal sympathetic tone and restoration of cortical perfusion (11). However, since sever
other manoeuvres such as acute hyperosmotic saline loading (12) or infusion of
pharmacological agents into the renal artery (13) are also able to increase
renal cortical blood-flow, other (functional) mechanisms may be operative as
well. The evaluation of such mechanisms does require a method of measuring ren
perfusion sufficiently flexible to demonstrate rapid changes in blood-flow. It
is obvious that under such circumstances the inert gas washout is preferable
above the clearance techniques since the latter rely too heavily on tubular
transport mechanisms.

Conclusions

The xenon washout technique seems to be an adequate method for assessing

renal perfusion. Although there is some doubt about the biological correlates
of the various components of the washout curve, there is considerable evidence
for localization of the first (fast-flow) component in the outer cortex of the
kidney. Bearing this in mind, it has become within reach to assess cortical
perfusion in various circulatory or renal disease states. However, there remains
a lot to be learned from the information produced by this technique. Not only
does this apply to the mechanisms responsible for a reduction in cortical flow,
but also and not in the least to the factors which govern xenon disappearance
from the kidney.

REFERENCES

1. Kety SS, Pharm. Rev. 3:1, 1951.

2. Andersen AM, Ladefoged J, Scand. J. clin. Lab. Invest. 19:72, 1966.

3. Thorburn GD et al. Circulat. Res. 13:290, 1963.

4. Dell RG et al. Circulat. Res. 32:71, 1973.

5. Ladefoged J, Scand. J. clin. Lab. Invest. 18:299, 1966.

6. Kolsters G, De Graaf CN, Neth. J. Med. 21:188, 1978.

7. Britton KE, Clin. Sci. 56:101, 1979.

8. Hollenberg NK et al. Sem. nucl. Med. 6:193, 1976.

9. Hollenberg NK et al. Amer. J. med. Sci. 261:232, 1971.

10. Hollenberg NK et al. Medicine 57:167, 1978.

11. De Leeuw PW, Birkenhäger WH, Hypertension 4:125, 1982.

12. Kolsters G, De bloedsomloop door de nieren bij essentiële hypertensie. The
    Rotterdam, 1976, p. 125.

BIOKINETICS OF Tc^{99m}-DTPA IN COMPARISON WITH HIPPURAN

Th. WHITE

The main reason for discussing the biokinetics of Tc^{99m}-DTPA in comparison with hippuran is, of course, that both substances are currently being used for gamma camera renography, also known as dynamic or functional renal imaging (1,2, 3,4,5,6). In addition, both substances can be used as indicators for clearance determinations (7,8,9). In either case, an understanding of their biokinetics is fundamental for correct clinical interpretation of the measurements.

Renography with hippuran is a classical diagnostic procedure, and it is a model example of how nuclear medicine can produce clinically important information on organ function quickly, easily, and with little discomfort to the patient. To an increasing extent, the original renographic single probe technique is now being superseded by gamma camera renography. The advantages of the gamma camera are obvious. The gamma camera eliminates one basic problem of the single probes, namely the localization of the kidneys, which mean that more quantitative data can be obtained. The gamma camera also makes possible more exact localization of functional disturbancies within the kidney and the outflow tract. In addition, the gamma camera provides some morphological information.

Hippuran can be labelled with different gamma-emitting isotopes of iodine. Hippuran labelled with iodine-131 is the classical indicator for single probe renography, and it has also been used for gamma camera renography. However, iodine-131 is not ideal for gamma camera imaging because of the relatively high energy of its photon. Iodine-131 gives poor image resolution. The sensitivity is lower than for technetium-^{99m}. As hippuran cannot easily be labelled with technetium, the remaining alternatives are either hippuran labelled with an isotope of iodine more suitable than iodine-131, or a technetium or other radio-nuclide compound suitable for renography.

Iodine-123 has a gamma ray energy spectrum similar to technetium-^{99m}, and hippuran labelled with iodine-123 produces good gamma camera images of the kidneys. I^{123}-hippuran is probably the best indicator for gamma camera renography. However, its use is hampered by high cost and limited availability. Iodine-123 is produced by cyclotrons, it has a half-life of 13 hours. Sometimes the user may be required to synthesize the hippuran from supplied iodine-123.

Instead, another kidney-seeking radiopharmaceutical, Tc^{99m}-DTPA, is often used for gamma camera renography. It is easily prepared from commercial kits, by addition of eluate from a technetium generator. DTPA is treated by the kidneys like EDTA. Both are so called GFR-substances, and they are chemically related (fig. 1). EDTA is chelating agent, a derivative of ethylene-di-amine. The letters EDTA stand for ethylene-di-amino-tetra-acetate. DTPA stands for diethylene-tri-amino-penta-acetate.

Hippuran and DTPA are excreted by the kidneys by different mechanisms. Both are filtered in the glomeruli. Hippuran is also secreted by the tubular epithelium. The renal clearance and extraction of hippuran are approximately four times greater than those of DTPA. So the choice between hippuran and DTPA is really a choice between different kidney functions to be studied. In many clinical situations disturbances in the renal handling of the two radiopharmaceutic.als seem to run in parallel, but this may not always be so.

In our department I^{131}-hippuran was used during several years for gamma camera renography. We then considered switching over to Tc-DTPA, and did a comparative study in which 37 patients were studied with both indicators (6). This may be illustrated by the gamma camera renograms obtained in one of the patients (fig. 1). Clearly, the two different radiopharmaceuticals produce curves of different shape. But it is also clear that each indicator can differentiate between a normal, and an abnormal pattern, such as the obstructive pattern, in the left kidney of fig. 1.

In general, the DTPA curves tend to be somewhat flatter, with less steep up-slope and down-slope. With DTPA, the peak of the curve may occur a little later than with hippuran. The renal parenchymal uptake of the two radiopharmaceuticals had approximately the same distribution between the kidneys, when the net uptake was calculated by substraction of background activity.

In order to quantitate the comparison of the curves obtained with the two radiopharmaceuticals, the time from injection to curve peak was determined in each renogram, and for each kidney the ratio between these two peak times was calculated. On average, the peak time was 13 per cent longer for DTPA (table 1)

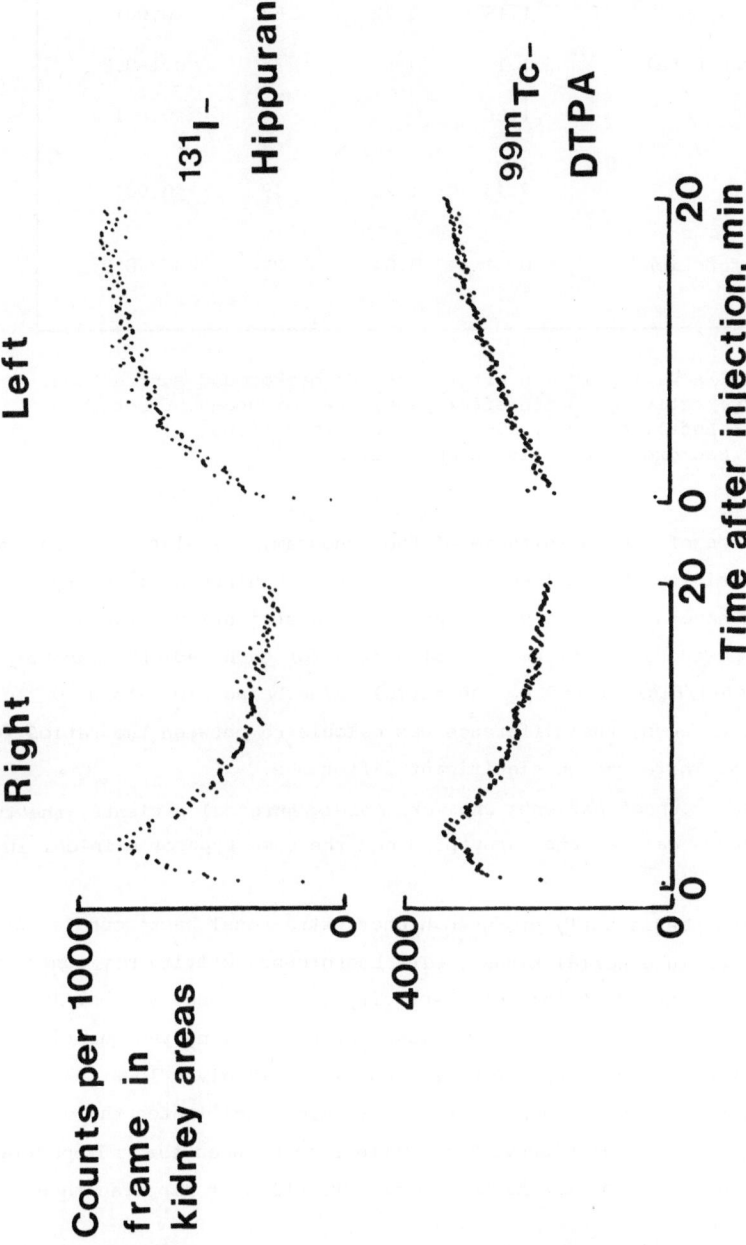

Fig. 1. Gamma camera renograms with I[131]-hippuran and TC-DTPA in a
34 year old man with stricture of the left ureter. Ordinates give
counts per 10 second frame in kidney areas.

Table 1. Gamma camera renography with I^{131}-hippuran and Tc^{99m}-DTPA in the same patients

	$\bar{x}$	SD	n	P(t-test)
Time to peak	1.13	0.22	54	<0.001
Diuresis (hippuran/DTPA)	1.13	0.54	34	0.1-0.2
Excretion ratio[1] (hippuran/DTPA)	1.66	0.36	49	<0.001
Excretion ratio[2] (hippuran/DTPA)	2.43	1.23	49	<0.001
Separate kidney function[3] (DTPA/hippuran)	0.01	0.04	27	0.2-0.3

[1] (Peak activity)/Activity 10 min after peak) No background-subtraction.
[2] (Peak activity)/Activity 10 min after peak). Background-subtraction.
[3] Right/(Right + Left). Activity 80-110 s after injection.
Corrected for background and tissue absorption.

The down-slope of the third phase of the renogram, calculated as peak acti ity divided by activity 10 min later, was steeper with hippuran in every single kidney which did have a renogram with a peak. The distribution between the kidneys of the net parenchymal uptake was calculated for each radiopharmaceutical as the ratio (Right)/Right + Left), the normal value being close to 0.50. In ea patient with two kidneys, the difference was calculated between the ratios for hippuran and DTPA. There was no significant difference.

Thus in this group of patients who were mainly surgical patients, the two indicators for gamma camera renography produced the same type of clinical information.

However, DTPA consistently produced higher extra-renal background activity than hippuran. Even in a normal kidney, DTPA background activity may contribute as much as about one third of the total activity in the kidney region. In a diseased kidney this proportion will increase further, making the quantificatio of net renal uptake less reliable. Hippuran consistently gives lower background activity, and higher organ-to-background ratio, which facilitates the quantific. tion in a poorly functioning kidney. This difference between the radiopharmaceuticals is a reflection of the higher renal extraction of hippuran than of DTPA.

If a laboratory for practical and economical reasons has to choose between I^{131}-hippuran and Tc-DTPA for routine gamma camera renography, the choice is difficult. The advantage of the lower background activity of hippuran must be weighed against the better image quality of Tc-DTPA. The choice is easy if I^{123}-hippuran is freely available. But even then the question remains unresolved whether there are situations where the different biological properties of hippuran and DTPA might make one indicator more suitable than the other, for the study of a particular clinical or physiological problem.

REFERENCES

1. Diffey BL, Hall FM, Corfield JR, J. nucl. Med. 17:352, 1976.

2. Kempi V, Persson RBR, Svensson L, In: Nuklearmedizin. 13. Int. Jahrestagun d. Ges. f. Nukl. med. 10-13 September 1975. Schattauer, Stuttgart, 1977.

3. Pors Nielsen S, Lehd Moller M, Trap-Jensen J, J. nucl. Med. 18:112, 1977.

4. Larsson I, Lindstedt E, Ohlin P, Strand SE, White T, Scand. J. clin. Lab. Invest. 35:517, 1975.

5. Macleod MA, Houston AS, Eur. J. nucl. Med. 6:183, 1981.

6. Bratt CG, Larsson I, White T, Scand. J. clin. Lab. Invest. 41:189, 1981.

7. Hilson AJW, Mistry RD, Maisey MN, Brit. J. Radiol. 49:794, 1976.

8. Klopper JF, Hauser W, Atkins HL, Eckelman WC, Richards P, J. nucl. Med. 13:107, 1972.

9. Tauxe WN, Dubovsky EV, Kidd T, Smith LR, Lewis R, Rivera R, Eur. J. nucl. 7:102, 1982.

DETERMINATION OF THE RADIOCHEMICAL PURITY OF HIPPURAN BY HPLC

G. PFEIFFER, I. BERANEK

INTRODUCTION

Hippuran, labelled with radioiodine is one of the most used radiopharmaceuticals in nuclear medicine. For the quantitative evaluation of renograms
and from the aspect of radiation dose, too, a good radiochemical purity of
hippuran is important.

Two different radioactive impurities are found in nearly all batches of
hippuran: radioiodide (I*) and labelled o-iodo-benzoic acid (o-I*-B). For the
radioiodide impurity there are 2 sources: a residue from the production procedure
itself (hippuric acid is labelled by isotopic exchange with radioiodide) or a
product from decomposition, especially in solutions of high specific activity
and of high radioactive concentration. The o-I-benzoic acid is an impurity of
the raw material hippuric acid, which will be labelled to a higher amount than
hippuric acid so that the amount of labelled o-I*-B is higher than the impurity
before labelling.

Methods

For the determination of the radiochemical purity of hippuran many of
methods are described in the literature, about 30 are listed in the papers of
Bögl (1). The European Pharmacopoeia (2) recommends paper chromatography in
butanol/acetic acid/water and thinlayer chromatography in benzene/acetic/acid/
water. These methods are very good in separating the impurities in hippuran,
but time consuming.

Producing I^{123}-labelled hippuran in our institute we attempted to find a
method, which gives the results of the radiochemical purity before delivering
the product and so we tried HPLC.

HPLC (high pressure or high performance liquid chromatography) is not yet
in general use for the quality control of radiopharmaceuticals. Two systems,
described in the literature, should be tested. Both use the reverse phase

system, but different solvent systems: methanol/water (3) and acetic acid/wat
(4,5).

The following parameters were tested: flow rate, injection volume and co
centration of the elution mixture. Our tests with the methanol system showed
good separation of radioiodide, hippuran and o-I-benzoic acid but the whole
procedure lasted more than one hour, using 12% methanol and a Biorad-column.

So we concentrated our work on the acetic acid system. First we looked f
the optimal concentration of acetic acid, determining the retention volume of
hippuran and o-I-B as function of acetic acid concentration or pH. Table I sh
the results.

TABLE 1

RETENTION VOLUMES AS FUNCTION OF ACETIC ACID CONCENTRATION

%	pH	ret.V.Hippuran	ret.vol. o-I-B
5	2.3	22.5 ml	85.7 ml
10	2.1	12.9 ml	48.3 ml
15	2.0	8.9 ml	30.1 ml
20	1.9	7.0 ml	20.3 ml
25	1.8	5.8 ml	14.7 ml
30	1.7	4.8	11.5 ml

High concentration of acetic acid or low pH reduces the time needed for the
analysis, but the separation is better with lower concentrations and higher p
As a compromise we found that 15% acetic acid will be the best for our purpos
to get exact results in a reasonable time. With this concentration we optimal.
the other parameters and used for the following experiments:
- Reverse phase column, Bio-Sil ODS-10 (Biorad), 250 x 4 mm
- 15% acetic acid
- 3 ml/min flow rate
- injection volume: 0.01 - 0.1 ml
- time for fractions: 42 s

With this system the retention volumes are:

- iodide : 4.0 - 4.5 ml
- hippuran: 9.0 - 10 ml
- o-I-B   : 30   - 33 ml

The time needed for a complete analysis is about 15 min.

Results

The first results of the radiochemical purity of 5 batches of I^{123}-hippuran analysed by HPLC and by the recommended
II.

TABLE II: I^{123}-hippuran: PC (paperchromatography) and HPLC

Batch	Radioiodide		Hippuran		o-I*-B.	
	PC	HPLC	PC	HPLC	PC	HPLC
97	1.0	1.4	98.4	97.9	0.6	0.7
98	0.6	0.7	99.0	98.6	0.4	0.7
99	0.7	1.0	98.5	97.9	0.8	1.1
100	0.7	0.9	98.8	98.5	0.5	0.6
101	0.6	0.9	98.8	98.3	0.6	0.7

The absolute values of the different impurities found with HPLC are slightly higher than with paper chromatography, but the correlation between these two methods is very good: the correlation factor is R = 0.9587, for o-I*-B R = 0.8656.

Summary

We tried HPLC for the determination of the radiochemical purity of hippuran. The method is rapid (about 15 min) and the results correspond very well with the pharmacopoea methods. Of course, some more comparative data must be collected before this method can be used for the routine control of hippuran in a production center.

REFERENCES

1. Heyde L, Stamm A, Schüttler Chr, Bögl W, Analytik radiochemischer Verunt-
   reinigungen in Radiopharmaka. STH-Berichte 15, 1979, 9, 1980, 5, 1981.

2. European Pharmacopoeia, suppl. vol. III, 199, 1977.

3. Bögl W, Stockhausen K, Censori M, Jahn M, Sander B, Untersuchungen über die
   radiochemische Reinheit einiger auf dem Markt befindlicher J-123/J-125/J-1:
   ortho-Jodhippurane. STH-Berichte 1, 1978.

4. Machulla HJ, Laufer P, Stöcklin G, Radioanalytical quality control of C-11
   F-18 and I-123-labelled compounds and radiopharmaceuticals. J. Radioanalyt
   Chem. 32:381, 1976.

5. De Jesus O, Djermouni B, Ache HJ, On the preparation of Br-80 labelled bio-
   molecules: solvent assisted labelling of hippuric acid via CF_3-Br-80-$KBrO_3$·
   technique. Intern. J. appl. Radiat. Isotop. 32:681, 1981.

TECHNETIUM COMPLEXES FOR RENAL SCINTIGRAPHY

P.H. Cox

INTRODUCTION

In the early 1950's renal scanning was first attempted using radioiodinated contrast media but these were soon superseded by mercurial complexes, notably chlormerodrin, labelled with ^{203}Hg or ^{197}Hg. These compounds had the advantage over contrast media that they became fixed in the renal cortex thus facilitating imaging and for many years they were the reagents of choice.

The first technetium compound to be used for renal imaging was an iron ascorbate complex developed by Harper in 1966 (1). About 8% of the administered activity was found to become fixed in the distal convoluted tubules the rest being excreted rapidly. Hauser et al (2) investigated the effect of differences in formulation on biodistribution in man and demonstrated these to be of a minor nature with about 6-8% of the administered dose remaining fixed in the kidneys between 4 and 24 hours post injection compared with 40 and 16% respectively for chlormerodrin. Iron preparations, however, can be irritant and with the development of simple one step labelling techniques using stannous ions as a reducing agent a number of technetium chelates have been prepared which are suitable for kidney imaging. Some of these are listed in table 1.

Halpern and Tubis et al (3,4,5) proposed the use of technetium penicillamine acetazolamide complex which showed a high degree of fixation in the renal cortex and later Halpern demonstrated that technetium penicillamine complexes without acetazolamide also showed an affinity for renal tissue. Tetracycline also complexes with technetium and becomes fixed in the kidney however, none of these complexes have come into common use.

It is well known that technetium phosphate complexes used for skeletal scintigraphy give excellent kidney images providing useful clinical information (6,7) but other chelates have become the reagents of choice for imaging. These can basically be divided into two groups:
- Those compounds such as DTPA EDTA and citrate which are excreted continuously by glomerular filtration (8,9,10). Of these the citrate complex (Solcocitran)

Table 1. Technetium complexes for renal imaging

> Iron ascorbate
>
> Glucoheptonate
>
> Gluconate
>
> DMSA
>
> DTPA
>
> Thiomalate (M.M.S.A.)
>
> Penicillamine acetazolamide
>
> Tetracycline
>
> EDTA
>
> Citrate
>
> Dextrose
>
> Aprotinin
>
> Phosphates
>
> Cysteine

has never been formally proposed as a renal imaging agent but in human stud in our hands it appears to give results comparable to DTPA.

- Those compounds such as DMSA (11,12) Dextrose (13) Thiomalic acid (14) and Glucoheptonate (15,16) which become fixed in the renal cortex primarily in proximal tubules.

Fig. 1 shows autoradiograms prepared of sections through rat kidneys showing, left: localization of DMSA in the cortex and right: citrate in both cortex and pyelum at 30 min post injection, to illustrate the fundamental diff ence between the two groups of compounds.

The kinetics of DTPA will be discussed elsewhere in this volume and the for it is not relevant to this presentation to consider this further. It is perhaps relevant to mention that it has been observed that variations in the formulation of stannous DTPA labelling kits does produce differences in bio-distribution and G.F.R. (17) This group of compounds are primarily used for function studies but can nevertheless also be used for scintigraphy.

An early scintigram produced a few minutes post injection will show act: ity primarily located in the renal cortex whilst a late scintigram prepared hour or later post injection will show a shift in activity to the pyelum. In this way the different regions of the kidney can be examined.

Fig. 2 shows the normal distribution of activity of technetium citrate complex (Solcocitran) in a normal kidney. The left hand scintigram is the ear.

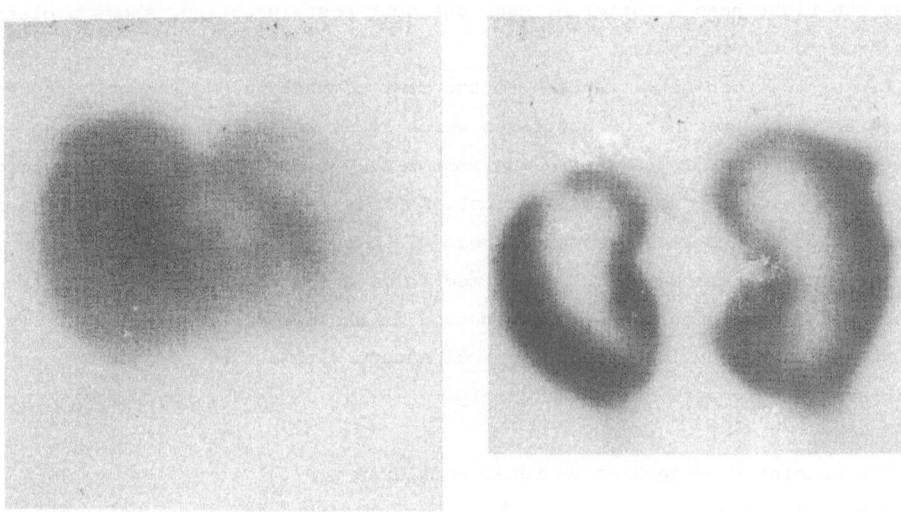

Fig. 1. Autoradiograms prepared of sections through rat kidneys showing DMSA and citrate.

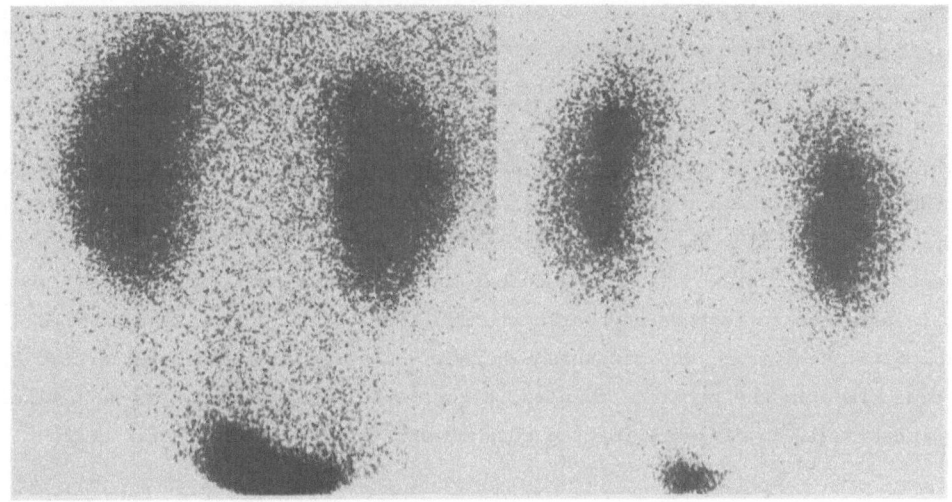

Fig. 2. The normal distribution of Tc-citrate in early and late scintigrams.

study prepared shortly after injection with activity in both cortex and pyelum whilst the right hand scintigram, made one hour post injection, shows a clear shift from cortex to pyelum.

Let us now turn our attention to the most commonly used reagents for rena scintigraphy, the technetium complexes which localize in the renal cortex. Of these glucoheptonate and DMSA are the most widely used and there is some contr versy as to which is the optimal reagent. DMSA is reported to show the highest concentration in the renal cortex whereas glucoheptonate has a faster and more complete blood-clearance which is claimed to give a higher kidney to backgroun ratio. Before examining the biodistribution of these compounds further it is perhaps useful to consider their chemical nature with a view to identifying possible structure activity relationships.

The chemistry of technetium renal complexes

The basic process involved in the formation of technetium complexes is th reduction of technetium from pertechnetate to a lower valency form which then complexes with the carrier to form a negatively charged ion. Formally, therefo it is incorrect to refer to Tc DTPA or glucoheptonate the correct terminology sodium Tc DTPA etc.

In the presence of excess stannous ions it is considered that Tc DTPA complexes are composed of Tc III bound to the carrier (18). Other complexes su as glucoheptonate have been shown to have technetium incorporated in the Tc V form. This may well explain why DTPA complexes are not bound in the renal cort whilst glucoheptonate and related substances are.

While elucidating the structure of technetium complexes in order to identify possible structure activity relationships we were able to establish (19,20), that two glucoheptonate ligands form a complex with one Tc V ion. The structure is shown in figure 3 and it is interesting to note that no tin is in corporated into the complex the stannous ions only act as electron donors. Thi phenomenon has been verified in a number of technetium complexes and as a resu it is possible to compare the structure and size of the molecules with their biological behaviour. The mechanism whereby glucoheptonate and related complex become fixed in the proximal tubules is not definitively known. The most likel explanation is an affinity for the sulphohydryl groups in the tubule cells.

Biodistribution studies

Let us now consider the biodistribution of the most commonly used reagent

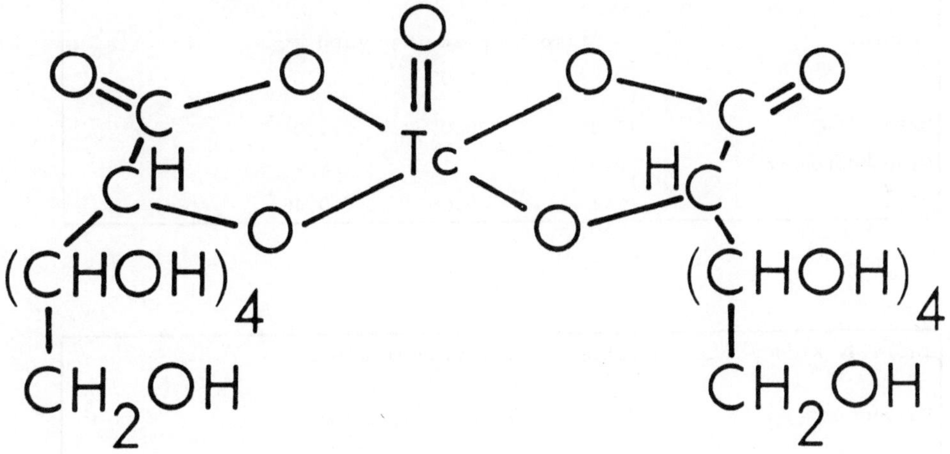

Fig. 3. The structure of Tc-glucoheptonate complex.

Table 2. Kidney / blood-ratios in the rat

Reagent	Time post injection	
	1 min	30 min
Glucoheptonate	8.6	22.5
DMSA	2.6	10.3
Aprotinin	6.4	30.1
Citrate	6.0	7.0
DTPA	5.7	7.0

to compare their performance with respect to the requirements for clinical imaging. First the kidney to blood-ratios. Table 2 shows the kidney to blood-ratios (% injected dose g/ml) of a number of reagents injected into rats, at human equivalent dose levels, shortly after injection and late, 30 min, post injection.

The increased concentration of glucoheptonate, DMSA and Aprotinin can clearly be seen whilst the lack of fixation of Citrate and DTPA is also evident. Aprotinin is a new reagent which will be refered to later. The glucoheptonate blood-clearance in the rat is faster than that of DMSA therefore the higher ratio

Table 3. Kidney uptake in the rat in relation to time post injection.
(% injected dose/organ)

Reagent	time hr post injection		
	0.5	1.0	2.0
DMSA	17.0	20.0	27.0
Glucoheptonate	8.8	9.1	8.7
DTPA	1.1	0.66	0.46

Table 4. Kidney / blood-ratios in relation to time.

Reagent	time hr post injection		
	0.5	1.0	2.0
DMSA	17.0	27.0	47.0
Glucoheptonate	44	93	160
DTPA	4.8	8.1	44

Table 5. Kidney to liver-ratios in the rat in relation to time.
(% dose g)

Reagent	time hr post injection		
	0.5	1.0	2.0
DMSA	8.7	17.0	28.0
Glucoheptonate	64	76	100
DTPA	13.0	13.0	12.0

Table 6. Radiation dose to the kidney in human subjects.

Reagent	rad /mCi
DMSA	0.62
Glucoheptonate	0.17
DTPA	0.042
Gluconate	0.21
Iron Ascorbate	0.27

of glucoheptonate is not surprising. Table 3 shows the actual kidney concentrations reached over a longer period of time where upon the higher concentration of DMSA becomes self evident. DTPA as might be expected shows no significant fixation.

The kidney to blood-ratios from the same group of animals are shown in table 4 where upon the effect of the faster blood-clearance of glucoheptonate can be clearly seen.

A further parameter worthy of consideration is the degree of uptake in the liver which can be of great significance in cases of renal malfunction. Table 5 shows the kidney to liver-ratios observed in this group of rats.

From this data it is possible to conclude that whilst glucoheptonate exhibits a considerably lower degree of accumulation in the kidney than DMSA the kidney to background-ratios are so much better that it should be the reagent of choice.

The biodistribution pattern is also reflected in the radiation dose to the kidney. Table 6. Once again glucoheptonate shows favourable characteristics.

The possible interrelationship between technetium complexes

At first sight there would appear to be little relationship between these various compounds to explain the differences in renal uptake and excretion. However, the elucidation of the structure of these compounds enables us to compare their biodistribution with molecular size. Fig. 4 shows the kidney uptake related to molecular weight which appears as a linear relationship in the rat. Similarly fig. 5 shows the distribution of a number of compounds in the rabbit which tends support to this proposition. Fig. 6 shows the distribution in humans of the preparations used to prepare fig. 4 and confirms the distribution patterns.

It would appear therefore that technetium chelates with an affinity for the renal cortex have similar biological properties which are influenced to some degree by the size of the molecule. In terms of kidney uptake to background-ratio, blood-clearance and radiation dosage sodium technetium glucoheptonate complex would appear to be the compound of choice. Fig. 7 shows a typical glucohepatonate scan with a normal right kidney and a left kidney showing diffuse inhomogenous uptake in hydronephrosis.

New developments - Aprotinin

Despite its high affinity for the renal cortex glucoheptonate, and indeed DMSA, show some degree of urinary excretion and there is a case for the develop-

38

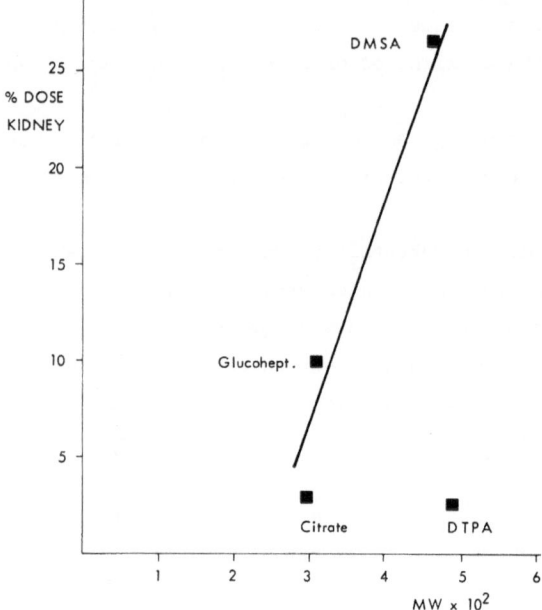

Fig. 4. Kidney uptake in the rat compared with the molecular weight of techn
tium complexes.

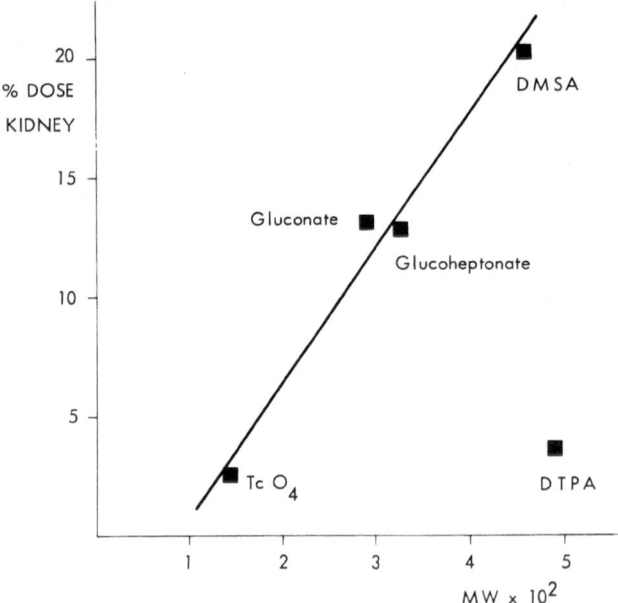

Fig. 5. Kidney uptake in the rabbit (calculated from ref. 16) compared with
molecular weight of technetium complexes.

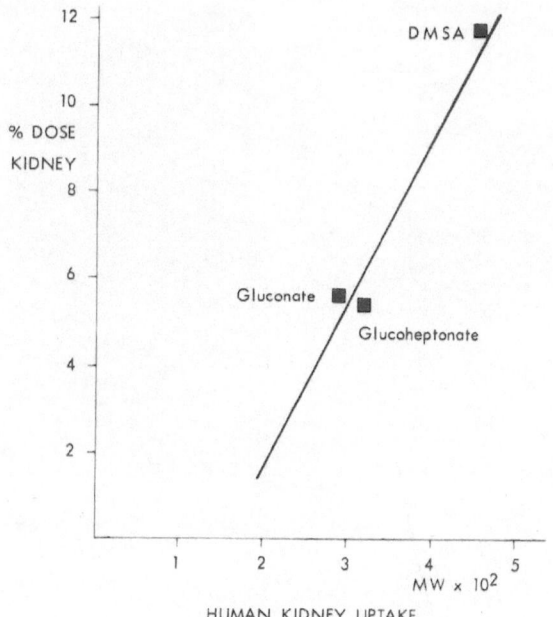

Fig. 6. Kidney uptake in humans compared with the molecular weight of technetium complexes.

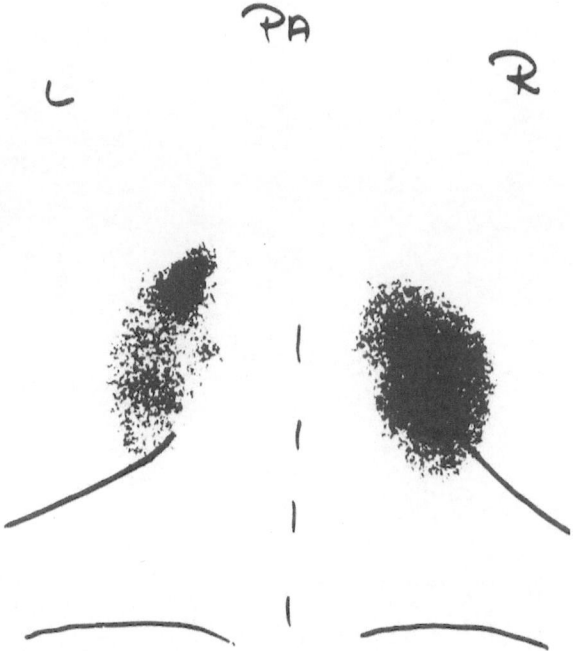

Fig. 7. Glucoheptonate scintigram of a normal right kidney and left with hydronephrosis.

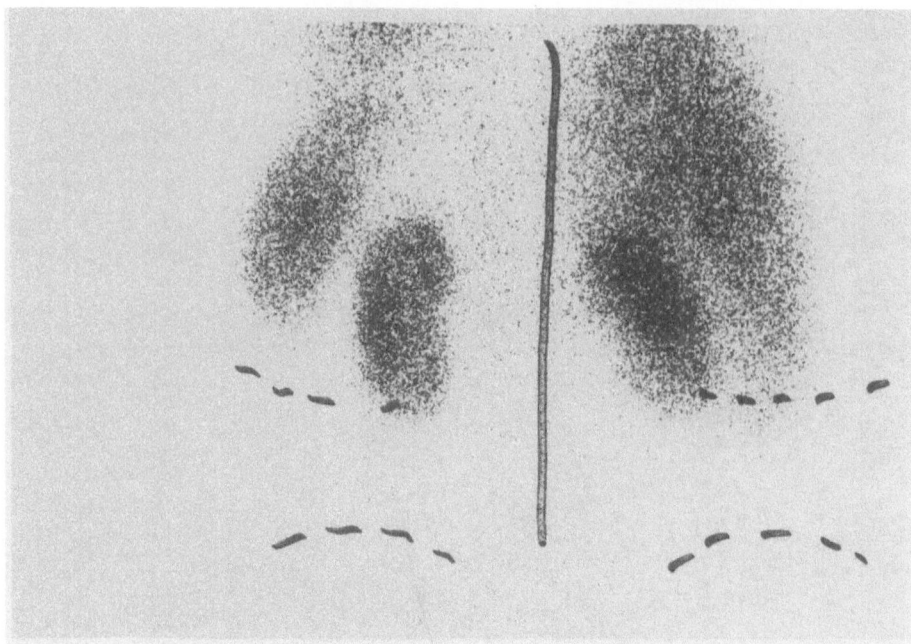

Fig. 8. Aprotinin scintigram 5 min post injection.

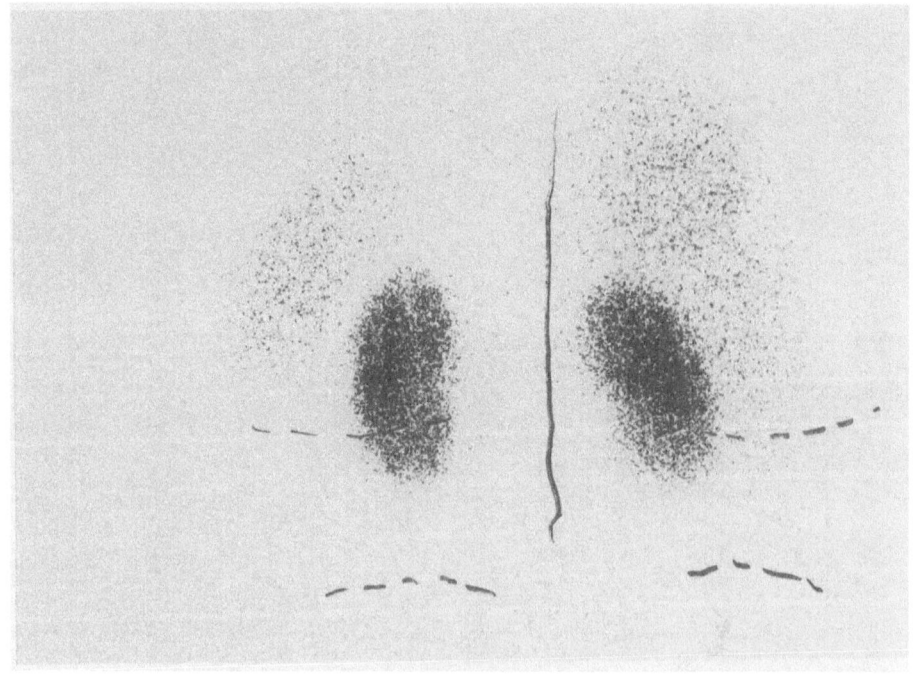

Fig. 9. Aprotinin scintigram 60 min post injection.

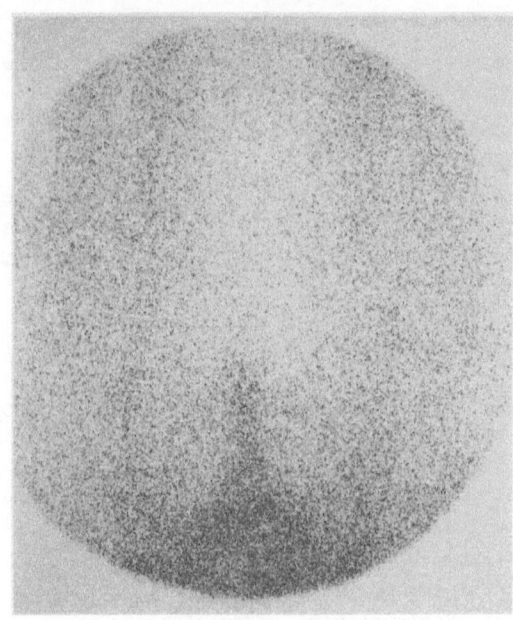

Fig. 10. Scintigram of lower abdomen to show lack of urine activity 60 min post injection.

ment of a more specific reagent. Aprotinin is a polypeptide, with a molecular weight of 6500, isolated from bovine lung with anti-enzyme properties. Villa and Lunghi (21) have developed a stannous labelling kit which provides a reagent with the following properties:

Blood T½	130 min
Cortex fixation in kidney	40% id 30 min p.i.
	60% id 3 hour p.i.
Urinary excretion	± 1% in the first 3 hours p.i.
Liver uptake	not measurable

Fig. 8 and fig. 9 show the renal uptake in a human subject at 5 and 60 min post injection, the liver- and spleenactivity is due to blood-background. Fig. 10 is a lower abdominal scintigram 60 min post injection to demonstrate the lack of urinary activity. This material is still in an early stage of development but appears to be very promissing.

REFERENCES

1. Harper PV et al. Technetium^{99m} iron complex. In: Radioactive Pharmaceutic
   USAEC Symposium, series No. 6, Andrews GE et al. (eds), 1966, p. 347-351.

2. Hauser W et al. Renal uptake of ^{99m}Tc iron ascorbic acid complex in man.
   Radiology 101:637, 1971.

3. Halpern SE et al. ^{99m}Tc penicillamine-acetazolamide complex. A new renal
   scanning agent. J. Nucl. Med. 13:45, 1972.

4. Halpern SE et al. ^{99m}TPAC a new renal scanning agent II evaluation in hum
   J. Nucl. Med. 13:723, 1972.

5. Tubis M et al. ^{99m}Tc- Penicillamine complexes. In: Radiopharmaceuticals.
   Society of Nuclear Medicine, New York, Subramanian G et al. (eds), 1975,
   p. 55-62.

6. Lavelle KJ et al. Renal hyperconcentration of ^{99m}Tc HEDP in experimental
   acute tubular necrosis. Radiology 131:491, 1979.

7. Glass EC et al. Immediate renal imaging and renography with ^{99m}Tc MDP to
   assess renal blood flow, excretory function and anatomy. Radiology 135:18
   1980.

8. Hauser W et al. Tc^{99m}DTPA a new reagent for brain and kidney scanning.
   Radiology 94:1369, 1970.

9. Klopper JF et al. Evaluation of ^{99m}Tc DTPA for the measurement of glomeru
   filtration rate. J. Nucl. Med. 13:107, 1972.

10. Agha NH et al. A new Tc^{99m} EDTA complex, production technique for renal
    studies. Int. J. appl. Radiat. Isot. 30:353, 1978.

11. Handmaker H et al. Clinical experience with Tc^{99m}DMSA a new renal imaging
    agent. J. Nucl. Med. 16:28, 1975.

12. Yee CA et al. Tc^{99m} DMSA renal uptake: influence of biochemical and physi
    logical factors. J. Nucl. Med. 22:1054, 1981.

13. Alvarex J et al. On a new radiopharmaceutical for kidney imaging. Int. J
    appl. Radiat. Isot. 25:283, 1974.

14. Hagan PL et al. ^{99m}Tc Thiomalic acid complex a non stannous chelate for
    renal scanning. J. Nucl. Med. 18:353, 1977.

15. Leonard JC et al. Renal cortical imaging and the detection of renal mass
    lesions. J. Nucl. Med. 20:1018, 1979.

16. Arnold RW et al. Comparison of technetium complexes for renal imaging. J.
    Nucl. Med. 16:357, 1975.

17. Carlsen JE et al. Comparison of four commercial Tc^{99m}Sn DTPA complexes us
    for the measurement of glomerular filtration rate. J. Nucl. Med. 21:126,
    1980.

18. Richard P, Steigman J, Chemistry of technetium as applied to radiopharma-
    ceuticals. In: Radiopharmaceuticals. Society of Nuclear Medicine, New Yor
    Subramanian G et al. (eds), 1975, p.23-35.

19. De Kieviet W, Tc glucoheptonate chemical structure and distribution.
    Proceedings III International Symposium on Radiopharmaceutical Chemistry,
    St. Louis, 1980, p. 136-137.

20. De Kieviet W, Recent developments in technetium chemistry. Nuk. Med. XX:2, 1981.

21. Villa M, Lunghi F, Private communication.

ENDOCRINOLOGY

THYROID PHYSIOLOGY : HORMONOGENESIS AND IODINE STORAGE

M.H. JONCKHEER

INTRODUCTION

The thyroid gland has a double specific role: iodine-dependent hormonogenesis and iodine-storage. The former is the most important one, but it depends
on the latter because the alimentary supply of iodine is either deficient on a
world-wide scale (1) or in any case intermittent. Hormonogenesis has been
extensively studied and its deviations have been used for diagnosis since about
four decades by means of radioactive iodine (RI) so extensively that it has been
assimilated in the minds of many practitioners as equal to thyroid function as a
whole. Up to now only indirect and cumbersome means were available for the study
of intrathyroidal stores (ITI) (2). The advent of the X-Ray Fluorescence method
(XFR) (3) makes this now possible as well for daily diagnostic purposes as for
physiopathological investigations (4). The relationship between the hypothalamus,
the hypophysis and thyroid function are also being used for diagnostic purposes
(5), although much is still to be understood concerning the fine regulation of
this system, and recent data cast new insights and interest in the autonomous
regulation of the thyroid cell (6,7). Thyroid hormones are synthetized and
stored within thyroglobulin (TG) (8), but the discovery of circulating TG in
health and disease (9) leads to interesting developments in the study of thyroid
function and adds to our diagnostic facilities.

In this presentation, we will recapitulate what is known about hormonogenesis, mostly in relation to the practice of nuclear medicine. We intend to
emphasize the recent advances in the understanding of thyroid physiology in
relation to stable iodine. A detailed discussion of the determination of thyroid
hormones in serum seems to be beyond the scope of this symposium and we consider
that aspecific radiopharmaceutical agents, such as ^{201}Tl for instance, do not
belong to these introductory remarks.

Thyroid hormonogenesis

The thyroid hormones are iodinated amino acids, occuring naturally as the

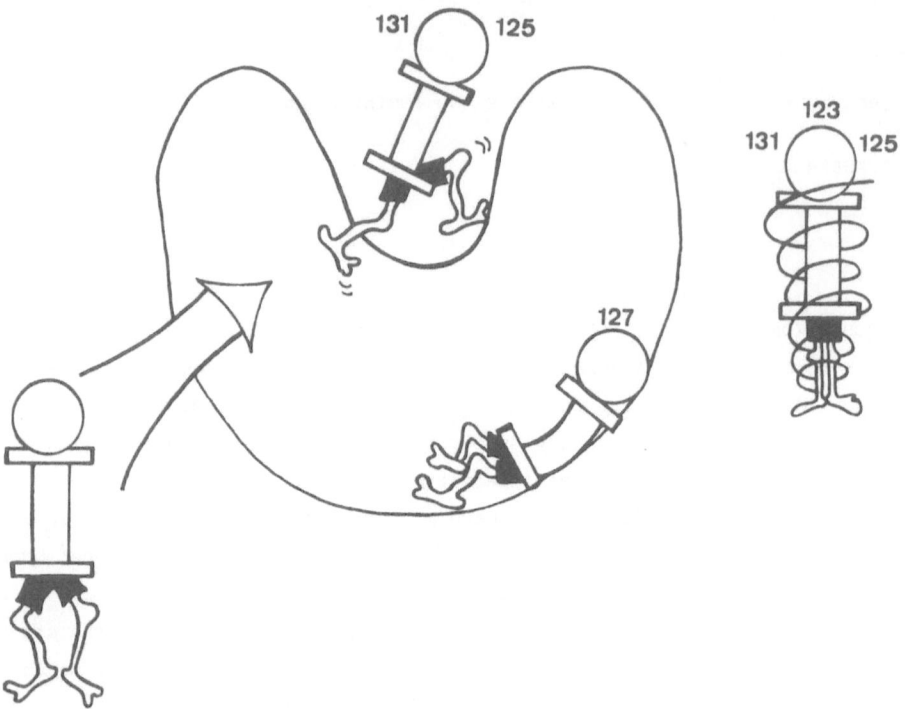

Fig. 1. Synoptic illustration of thyroidal iodine pathways. NB: I-127=stable iodine. See text for explanation.

L-isomers: L-tetraiodothyronine (L-thyronine, T4), 65% iodine by weight and L-triiodothyronine (T3), 58% iodine by weight. They are synthesized within thyroglobulin, where they are stored. Thyroglobulin can be removed from the follicular lumen by a process of endocytosis. T4 and T3 are released by proteolysis into the circulation. At this same step of thyroid metabolism, some iodide is reintroduced into the cycle, some thyroglobulin is released into circulation, even in normal circumstances, and some iodine is lost ("iodide leak"), under an unknown organic form, part of which could be thyralbumin (10). A schematic representation of the iodine pathways is shown in fig. 1. Uptake, organification, release under hormonal form and leak of iodine have been extensively studied by means of RI and clinical applications deriving from these studies are ubiquitou

Enhanced iodide-leak can be found in many pathological situations, mainly in autoimmune disease of the thyroid, such as atrophic autoimmune thyroiditis, Hashimoto's disease and Graves' disease (11). When ^{131}I is administrated in these cases, an abnormally high PBI-131 can be measured after 24 hours, most of

TABLE 1

Scanning Agent	Activity Administrered	Local Dose (Thyroid)	Whole Body Dose
I 131 (NaI)	50 µCi	65 rads	23 mrads
I 125 (NaI)	50 µCi	41 rads	20 mrads
Tc 99 (NaTcO$_4$)	1 mCi	.1 rads	10 mrads
I 123	100 µCi	1-2 rads	Very small
X-ray Fluorescence	0 µCi	.017 rads	0 mrads

it being non-butanol extactable (NBEI). We feel nevertheless that this measurement has become obsolete in nowadays clinical practice.

We are also of the opinion that routine studies of iodine kinetics by means of RI, ^{123}I included, is not warranted anymore and should be reserved for special situations. This for many reasons. The physical properties of ^{131}I and ^{125}I result in a relatively high radiation burden (table 1) and are not optimal for external detection; ^{123}I is too expensive from a cost/benefit point of view. They add unnecessary, although minor, discomfort to the work-up of a thyroid problem. Falsely low turnover rates can be found in cases of iodine contamination which is very often unsuspected and unknown, as well as under the influence of a substitution therapy with l-T4. Antithyroid medication gives unpredictable results of the turnover studies. In earlier days, the RI uptake was represented under the form of a true curve, determined by at least three points, giving some consistency for its interpretation. It has become customary to replace this "curve" by a single determination at 24 hours which is of course conceptually wrong and can be misleading. Indeed, fast turnover rates can result in a rapid clearance of radioactivity from the thyroid and will only be detected if a high PBI-131 is found at that time. Again the true hormonal form of this high PBI-131 will only be shown if the proportion of NBEI-131 is calculated, a cumbersome procedure. Furthermore, fast turnover rates without hyperthyroidism are the rule when the total amount of functioning thyroid tissue has been reduced by disease or after surgery.

By far the most powerful argument against the routine use of RI in the diagnosis of dyshormonogenesis is the fact that the net result, i.e. the thyr state of the patient, can be estimated with great accuracy by a careful clini examination, supported by appropriate measurements of circulating thyroid hormones. In our department, ^{131}I investigations are limited to those hyper-thyroid patients who are candidates for ^{131}I treatment.

For the imaging of the thyroid gland, RI can advantageously be replaced $^{99m}TcO_4$. (Tc) from the point of view of ease and comfort to the patient, radi tion burden and costs. Tc may be considered to be a specific pharmacological agent as its uptake depends upon the same factors as those of RI uptake. Although some evidence has been presented that organification might take plac (12), it is generally admitted that Tc does not follow the I pathway further than the uptake step. It follows that the uptake (and therefore the visualiza tion of the gland) will be influenced in the same circumstances as those vali for RI: iodine contamination, T3-suppression, TSH-stimulation, etc. It follow that the images obtained with these two types of radiopharmaceuticals are bas ally different: a functional image of uptake with Tc and a functional image o the organification process with RI. These differences may account for the dis crepancies sometimes described between the scintigraphy affectuated with thes two agents in the same patient (13).

A Tc uptake index has been advocated as a practical way to study the fir step of hormonogenesis (14). The same theoretical objections can be made as i the case of the RI uptake test. Nevertheless, because we use a pinhole collim tor and a gamma camera for imaging the thyroids with Tc, we complete this st routinely with a variant of the proposed method. It only takes 3 min more tha the examination time, positioning and data-processing included, and we found to yield useful indicative, although not essential, information. Hyperthyroid and simple goitres due to iodine deficiency present with high indices whereas low index may point towards iodine contamination or thyroid suppression.

Stable iodine and thyroid function

Endemic goitre due to iodine deficiency is a world-wide problem (1) and many developed countries, iodine has been supplemented in the diet with remar

able success. Confirmation of this beneficial prevention has been lately confirmed a contrario in The Netherlands. Since many years, iodine is supplemented in
bread in this country with a decrease in the incidence of goitre as a result.
For some time anyhow, the prevalence seemed to rise again and this could be
related to a lesser consumption of bread (15), demonstrating the efficacity of
the health measure that had been taken.

The normal thyroid gland contains about 9 mg iodine as measured in vivo in
man (4) and the normal concentration, as measured by chemical means is 0.325 mgI
+ 0.045 per g/tissue (16). When the iodine concentration decreases to a level
lower than 0.250 Img g/tissue, the TG molecule undergoes steric distortion,
resulting in inadequate synthesis of the hormones (17). We recently found (18)
that below the amount of 2 to 3 mg ITI, the hyman thyroid gland becomes in-
efficient and data that will be presented at this symposium confirm that normal
thyroid function is disrupted at an iodine concentration of about 0,2 mg I
g/tissue.

It is thus obvious that a minimal amount of iodine is necessary for normal
thyroid homeostasis. 0.075 mg I are needed daily, but the mean intake in most
non endemic areas of the world where iodine is not supplemented (in Belgium e.g.),
is only 0.100 mg (19,17). If one takes into account the obligatory urinary losses
(normal iodide clearance amounts to 30-50 ml/min) (8) and also the fact that
alimentary intake (essentially seafood and milk) (20,21) is intermittent, it is
also obvious that iodine storage is of paramount importance.

By means of the XRF technique, it was possible to confirm in vivo in man
that about 2/3 of sporadic goitres contain less ITI than normal glands, that the
ITI undergoes seasonal variations with a maximum in April and a minimum in September (22) and that the stable iodine pool can be restored by intermittent small
doses of iodide (23), A beneficial effect of small intermittent doses of iodide
(2 mg twice a month) on size of the goitre and restoration of normal hormone
concentrations could be shown recently by Ermans (24). It should nevertheless
not be forgotten that other factors than iodine deficiency most certainly are at
the origin of sporadic goitre (25), such as e.g. thiocyanate (26) or possibly
antibodies (27).

On the other hand, the administration of stable iodine may have a deleter-
ious effect upon thyroid function. Excess iodide provokes an inhibition of
iodine organification, a phenomenon known as the Wolff-Chaikoff effect (28),
depending upon the relative concentration of iodide on both sides of the thyroid
cell membrane. In normal glands, there usually follows an escape from this block.

On other occasions, excess iodide can induce goitre, hypothyroidism or hyperthyroidism (29,30) and it is generally accepted, though not totally proven, tha
this untoward effect of iodide occurs in already diseased glands (8). This inhibition or activation as an explanation for some human thyroid disorders,
relied so far upon indirect evidence or animal and in vitro studies. With the
XRF method it is now possible to demonstrate a direct relationship between the
ITI and some cases of hyperthyroidism (31) as well as to explain cases of dys-
thyroidism due to iodine-containing drugs (32,33). It can therefore be conclude
that the assessment of ITI can be of value in daily practice.

There still remains controversy as to the concentration at which plasma
iodide produces its inhibitory effect. As early as 1949, Stanley (34) showed
that an intake of 1 mg I was not inhibitory, whereas 2 mg probably was. The
doses refered to in this section for the treatment of sporadic goitre (intermittent administration of 1 to 2 mg I weekly or twice a month) demonstrated a
beneficial effect. Nevertheless, recent observations in our department (35) sho
that the administration of 1 mg or 2 mg I once a week to normal volunteers
produces a temporary inhibition of thyroid hormone secretion followed by a
spontaneous escape without any clinical expression. It could also be shown that
this effect was probably independent from the pituitary-thyroid axis, thus representing an autonomous regulation mechanism of the thyroid cell, but that it
was modulated by the stable iodine pool. It follows that an inhibitory dosis of
iodide will be very difficult to define.

Summary

Thyroid function is directly related to iodine metabolism. Iodine is taken
up, organified under the form of hormones that are subsequently either secreted
or stored. The whole process can be studied by means of RI, the storage functio
with much difficulty. It is felt that from a diagnostic point of view, the use
of RI should be reserved to special situations.

Nuclear medicine procedures allow to obtain different functional images of
the thyroid: an uptake image by means of Tc, an organification image by means o
RI and a storage image by means of the XRF method.

This last method has proven to be very useful for the study of the effect
of stable iodine upon thyroid function and holds much promise as a daily investigation tool.

REFERENCES

1. Dunn JT, Medeiros-Neto GA, Endemic goitre and cretinism: continuing threats to world health. PAGO, Washington, Scientific Publication, 1975, p. 292.

2. DeGroot LJ, Kinetic analysis of iodine metabolism. J. clin. Endocr. 26:149, 1966.

3. Hoffer PB, Jones WB, Crawford RB, Gottschalk A, Fluorescent Thyroid Scanning: a new method of imaging the thyroid. Radiology 90:342, 1968.

4. Jonckheer MH, Deconinck F, X-Ray-Fluoresence determination of stable iodine in the thyroid gland: a review. Acta clin. belg. 1982 (In press).

5. DeGroot LJ, Cahill GF, Odell WD et al. Endocrinology, Vol. 1, Grune & Stratton (eds), New York, 1979.

6. Yukimura Y, Ikejiri K, Kojima A, Yamada T, Effect of excess iodide secretion in normal or hypophysectomized rats treated with graded doses of thyroid hormone. Endocrinology 99:541, 1976.

7. Trost BN, Buchli R, Osterwalder HJ, Kohler H, Konig MP, Studer H, The handling of moderately excessive iodide loads by normal and goitrous human thyroid glands. J. Mol. Med. 4:167, 1980.

8. DeGroot LJ, Stanbury JB, The thyroid and its diseases. John Wiley and Sons, New York, 1975.

9. Van Herle AJ, Vassart G, Dumont JE, Ccntrol of thyroglobulin synthesis and secretion. New Engl. J. Med. 301:307, 1979.

10. Jonckheer MH, Thyralbumin as a true thyroid protein. Thesis, Brussels, 1973.

11. Bastenie PA, Ermans AM, Thyroiditis and thyroid function, Pergamon Press, G.B. 1972.

12. Burke G, Halks A, Silverstein GE, Hilligoss M, Comparative thyroid uptake studies with 131-I and 99m-TcO^4. J. clin. Endocr. Metab. 34:630, 1972.

13. Balachandran S, Sayle BA, Discordant thyroid nodule images with pertechnetate at 30 minutes and 3 hours. Clin. Nucl. Med. 3:340, 1978.

14. Selby JB, Buse MG, Gooneratne NS, Moore DO, The Anger camera and the per-technetate ion in the routine evaluation of thyroid uptake and imaging. Clin. Nucl. Med. 4:233, 1979.

15. Querido A, Tan WD, Relating goitre incidence to urinary iodine excretion. Ann. Endocr. (Paris), 42:39A, 1981, (abstract).

16. Reinwein D, Durrer HA, Meinhold H, Iodine thyroxine (T4), triiodothyronine (T3), 3,3',5'-triiodothyronine (rT3), 3,3'-dioiothyronine (T2) in normal human thyroids. Effect of excessive iodine exposure. Horm. Met. Res. 13:456, 1981.

17. Ermans AM, Kinthaert J, Camus M, Defective intrathyroidal iodine metabolism in non-toxic goitre: inadequate iodination of thyroglobulin. J. clin. Endocr. Metab. 28:1307, 1968.

18. Jonckheer MH, Vanhaelst L, Deconinck F, Michotte Y, Atrophic Autoimmune Thyroiditis. Relationship between the clinical state and intrathyroidal iodine as measured in vivo in man. J. clin. Endocr. Metab. 53:476, 1981.

19. De Crombrugghe B, Beckers C, De Visscher M, General aspects of iodine metabolism in sporadic goitre. Acta endocr. (Khb) 42:300, 1963.

20. Aabach HS, Jodutskillesle i urin, i relasjon til forskjellige viktige fodemidler. Intern. Rapport F-365, Forsvarets Forskningsinstitutt. Norwegi Defence Research Establishment, Norway, 1976.

21. Grayson RR, Factors which influence the radioactive iodine uptake test. Amer. J. Med. 28:397, 1960.

22. Jonckheer MH, Coomans D, Broeckaert I, Van Paepegem R, Deconinck F, Season variation of stable intrathyroidal iodine in nontoxic goitre disclosed by X-ray fluoresence. J. Endocr. Invest. 1981 (In press).

23. Jonckheer MH, Deconinck F, X-stralen fluorescentie: vier jaar ervaring. Nucl. Gen. Bull. 3:118, 1981.

24. Ermans AM, Verelst J, Acute effects of supra-physiological doses of iodine in the human being: management of non-toxic goitre. J. Mol. Med. 4:199, 19:

25. Henneman G, Non-toxic goitre. Clin. Endocr. Metab. 8:167, 1979.

26. Bourdoux P, Delange F, Gerard M, Mafreta M, Hanson A, ERmans AM, Evidence that Cassava ingestions increases thyrocyanate formation: a possible etiolic factor in endemic goitre. J. Clin. Endocr. Metab. 46:613, 1978.

27. Drexhage HA, Battazzo GF, Doniach D, Bitensky L, Chayen J, Growth-stimulat. immunoglobulins (TGI) contribute to goitre formation. Ann. Endocr. (Paris) 42:14A, 1981, (abstract).

28. Wolff J, Chaikoff IL, Plasma organic iodide as a homeostatic regulator of thyroid function. J. biol. Chem. 174:555, 1948.

29. Wolff J, Iodide goitre and the pharmacologic effects of excess iodide. Ame: J. Med. 47:101, 1969.

30. Braverman LE, Ingbar SH, Changes in thyroidal function during adaption to large dosis of iodide. J. clin. Invest. 42:1216, 1963.

31. Jonckheer MH, Deconinck F, Swaenepoel L, Upon the importance of different-iating between two forms of hyperthyroidism by means of X-ray fluorescence scanning. In: Thyroid Research VIII. Australian Academy of Sciences, Stockligt JR, Nagataki S (eds), Canberra, Australia, 1980, p. 637.

32. Jonckheer MH, Iatrogenic hypothyroidism. In: Recent progress in diagnosis and treatment of hypothyroid conditions. Excerpta Medica, Congress Series, 529, Bastenie PA, Bonnijns M, Vanhaelst L, (eds),Amsterdam, 1980, p. 15.

33. Jonckheer MH, Amiodarone and the thyroid gland - a review. Acta cardiol. 36:199, 1981.

34. Stanley MM, The direct estimation of the rate of thyroid hormone formation in man. The effect of the iodide ion on thyroid iodine utilisation. J. clir Endocr. Metab. 9:941, 1949.

35. Jonckheer MH, Michotte Y, Van Steirteghem AC, Deconinck F, Inhibition of thyroid secretion by physiological doses of iodide in the normal human thyroid gland, modulated by intrathyroidal iodine stores. Advances on Thyroid Hormones, Pisa 1982:42, 1982, (abstract).

A SIX COMPARTMENT MODEL FOR THE STUDY OF EARLY KINETICS OF THYROID
TRAP IN HUMANS - METHODOLOGY AND RESULTS

J.P. BAZIN, P. FRAGU, R. DI PAOLA

INTRODUCTION

The possibility of using sophisticated computer systems, especially concerning calculating power and man-machine dialogue, in a clinical setting is the
basis for a new surge in model analysis in nuclear medicine. The combination of
this analysis with self-modeling type methods, used for automating the processing of dynamic examinations (1,2), should lead to their development in parallel
with the increasing importance of physiological and metabolic studies (3).
Recently, the group of Berman (4) has introduced a new conversational version
of the well known Saam program. To our knowledge this software was designed for
large computer systems and has not yet been installed in the more modest systems,
generally used in clinical practice. The conversational software, Clinmod that
we have developed, can be used for the compartmental analysis of data acquired
in dynamic scintillation camera studies. The software was written in Fortran and
installed in an Infogram* computer. We described the method used in our laboratory
for processing dynamic studies with compartmental models and the results obtained in a comparison of early iodine and technetium kinetics.

Materials and methods

Data acquisition and processing were performed with a gamma camera computer
system (5). The methodology has been previously described (6). Dynamic thyroid
studies were performed for 60 to 150 min following an intravenous injection of
37 to 185 MBq (1 to 5 mCi) of Tc^{99m} or radioiodine. Before injection, the
syringes containing the isotopes were counted in a neck phantom at 8 to 10 cm
from the neck of patients in supine position. Several list mode acquisitions
(maximum 450,000 counts) were performed during the first 30 min of the test.
Subsequently, 50,000 counts list mode acquisitions were performed. Pertechne-

* Informatek (France)

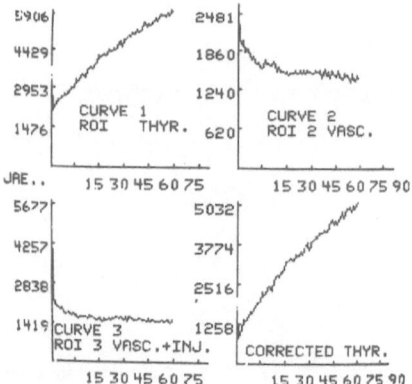

Fig. 1. Curves obtained into three different ROI. The corrected thyroid curve is the result of the subtraction curve 2 (vascular ROI) from curve 1 (thyroid ROI) after subsequent normalizations.

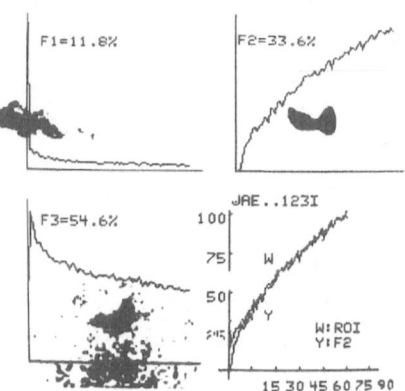

Fig. 2. F1,F2 and F3 are dynamic components and spatial structures extracted from the dynamic images sequence by means of factor analysis. F1, F2 and F3 are respectively: injection, thyroid and vascular components. W and Y are respective ly curves obtained with the ROI method and factor analysis.

tate and iodine blood radioactivities were determined at 2, 5, 8, 18, 30 and 60 min. For the 150 min studies, three additional points were collected at 90, 120 and 150 min. Dynamic curves were initially obtained from the list mode acquisitions for selected regions using the region of interest (ROI) technique, (fig. 1)

Vascular background was corrected by subtracting counts in equal sized area located near the thyroid gland from counts in the thyroid region itself. The uptake curves were obtained by reference to the standard after correction for

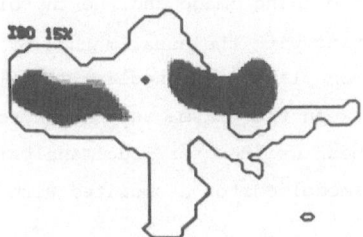

Fig. 3. Superimposition of injection and thyroid factors.

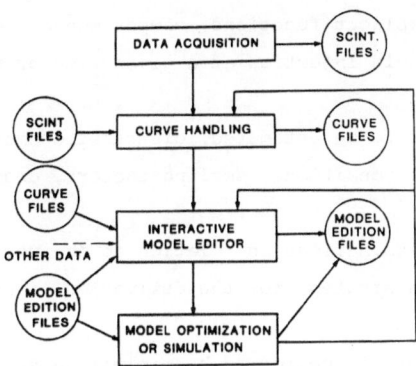

Fig. 4. CLINMOD. Interactive system for model analysis.

radioactive decay.

Correction using vascular background subtraction is generally insufficient because of the impossibility of choosing a ROI exclusively representing the contribution of blood-activity to the thyroid gland. From our point of view the initial points of the corrected thyroid curve are not satisfactory from a physiological stand point because at time 0, the value of thyroid activity is not equal to zero. This is not surprising as the ROI method cannot take into account the exact vascular contribution inside the thyroid. To avoid this difficulty we have used a method developed in our laboratory based on the factor analysis of dynamic structures (3). This method leads to the automatic resolution of the problem of superimposition without having to draw ROI. Fig. 2 shows factors F1, F2, F3 and the corresponding factorial images obtained for the same patient as above. It enables the results furnished by the two methods to be compared (fig. 2

bottom right). With this method the thyroid curve pass through zero.

Fig. 3 shows the superimposition of the injection factor delineated by the isocount 15 percent of the maximum corresponding image and the thyroid factor, emphasizing the impossibility of correcting with the usual method of ROI. It is important to remember that this correction plays a not negligible role in the determination of exchange parameters between the plasma and the thyroid gland.

The Clinmod software (fig. 4) has been written for model analysis purposes It is mainly composed of an interactive model editor associated with curve file and model edition files management.

The editor is linked with data acquisition and optimization programs. Its functions are mainly:

a. The definition of the model used: explicit functions, compartmental model wi constant coefficients and with a single injection at a given time or model w: an input function, etc.

b. The choice of parameters (imposed or to be estimated) distributed among 8 classes: exchange constants, initial conditions, scaling factors, undirectional clearance (open models)..

c. The description of experimental determinations in relation to the model.

d. The introduction of the optimization strategy for the estimation of unknown parameters.

The estimation of unknown parameters is performed by minimizing the normal ized least squares criterion:

$$Q = \frac{1}{m} \sum_{j=1}^{m} \frac{\sum_{i=1}^{n_j} w_{ij} (y_{ij} - \hat{y}_{ij})^2}{\sum_{i=1}^{n_j} w_{ij}}$$

y_{ij}: point "i" curve "j" $\hat{y}_{ij}$: model solution w_{ij}: weight

m : number of curves n_j : number of experimental points of the curve "j"

This criterion enables the contribution of m measurements to be balanced, of which each includes n_j experimental points. w_{ij} is the weight of the point y_{ij} and $\hat{y}_{ij}$ is the solution furnished by the model for the same point. The criterio Q is minimized by combining an adaptive Monte-Carlo method (7) and the simplex

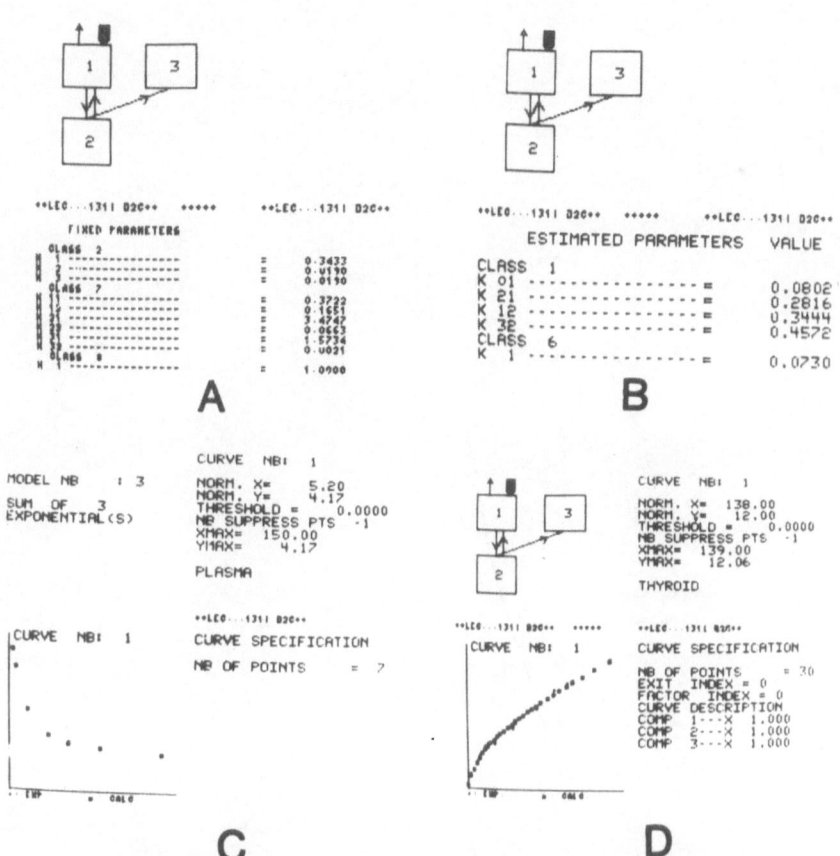

Fig. 5. A: open 3-compartment model and fixed parameters; B: estimated parameters; C: fitting of the plasma activity curve (input function to compartment 1); D: fitting of the thyroid curve with the open 3-compartment model. These four pictures are the direct output on the colour TV monitor of the CLINMOD software.

	A	B	C
Q	0.416	0.466	0.396
k_{01} (mn^{-1})	0.08	0.04	0.61
k_{21} (mn^{-1})	0.28	0.53	0.82
k_{12} (mn^{-1})	0.34	0.50	0.58
k_{32} (mn^{-1})	0.46	0.17	0.37
R (ml.mn^{-1})	73.	64.	143.

TABLE 1 . COMPARISON OF SOLUTIONS
OBTAINED BY USING DIFFERENT STRATEGIES:
A) AND B) FOR TWO DIFFERENT INITIALISA-
TIONS; C)FOR A CONSTRAINED CONSTANT k_{01}.

60

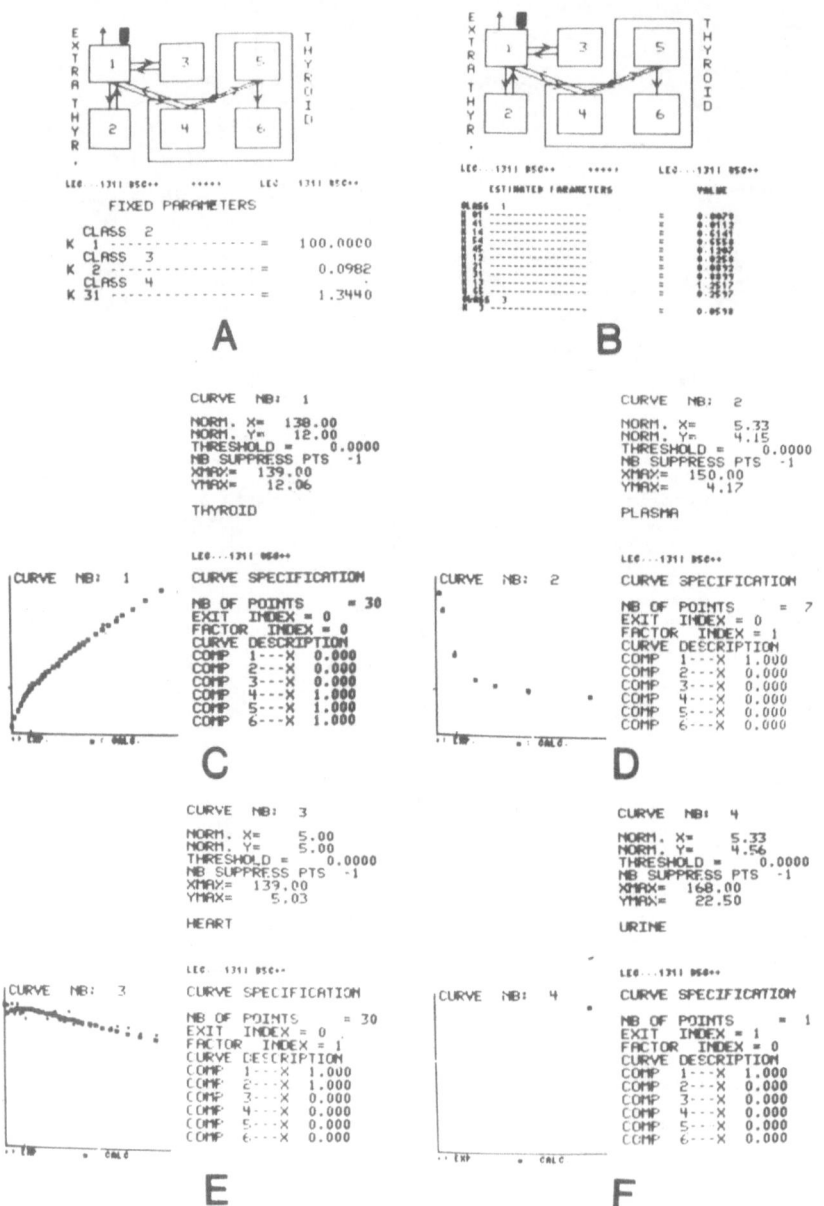

fig. 6. 6-compartment model. A: fixed parameters; B: estimated parameters; C: to F simultaneous fitting of experimental data.

method as described by Olsson (8).

The comparison of early iodine and technetium kinetics was initially performed with models described in the literature (9,10), especially the open 2 or 3 compartment thyroid models with a plasma input function (fig. 5). This input was fitted with a 3 exponential function and the estimations obtained were used as fixed parameters in fitting the 3 compartment open system. Modifying the initializer of the iterative process in the Monte Carlo method enabled solutions A and B to be obtained. They are different (table 1) and lead to perfect fits.

The estimation of the constant K_{01}, which in this model does not participate in the fitting of extra-thyroid measurement, is very low in both cases. By fixing a value to the exit rate constant $K_{01} = 0.61$ (K_{14} in the 6-compartment model; fig. 6), we obtained an estimation of the parameters (table 1-C) completely different from the others (A and B). Fitting of the thyroid curve obtained in these conditions gives a Q value lower than that in examples A and B. These results emphasize the great instability of the estimates with the open compartment model. This is why we have used a 6-compartment model for the study of the early thyroid trap. The 6 compartment model (fig. 6) has been described in more detail (elsewhere) (6). Compartments 1 to 3 are introduced to take into account all the extrathyroid iodide spaces. Compartments 4 to 6 are thyroid compartments which are defined in relation to the 3 compartment model described by Wollman and Reed (11). Compartment 6 is the organification compartment.

By giving a compartmental structure to the extrathyroid spaces we introduce a physiological constraints on parameters $_{41}$ and $_{14}$ that both contribute to simultaneous fits of the plasma, thyroid, cardiac curves and urinary excretion (fig. 6).

Results and discussion

The main advantage of the early kinetic study is to obtain more information about the retention of iodide in the gland than with the conventional clearance in which the radioiodide released soon after its retention by the thyroid is not taken into account. The 6 compartment model assesses the unidirectional (R_{41}) and irreversible (R_{65}) thyroid clearances, the rapid return of trapped iodide to the plasma (λ_{14}) and the sizes of the thyroidal iodide pools (V_4 and V_5).

Iodide kinetics: Fig. 7 summarizes the results of the thyroidal part of the 6 compartment model after intravenous injection of radioiodine.

In euthyroid patients, the two intrathyroid iodide compartment sizes (V_4

62

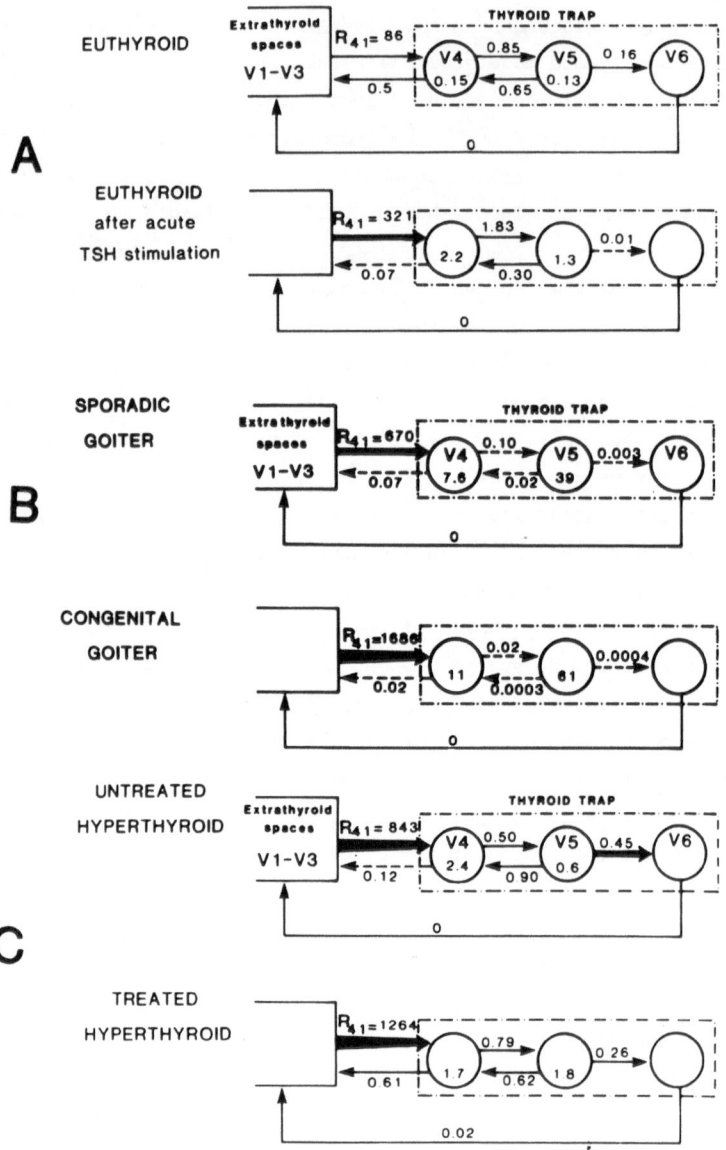

Fig. 7. Summary of the results obtained with the 6 compartment model: $R_{41} = \lambda_{41}$ (ml.min^{-1}); the other parameters are: λ_{ij} transfert constants (min^{-1}) and size of V_4 and V_5 (liter of plasma equivalent volume).

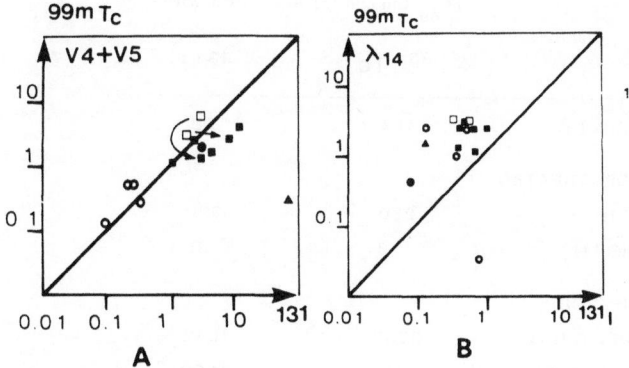

Table 2   EARLY KINETICS OF THYROID STRAP :
ESTIMATES OF THE IODIDE CLEARANCES
AND THE IODIDE LOSS

	R_{41} ml.min^{-1}	R_{65}^{**} ml.min^{-1}	$R_1 = \dfrac{R_{14}}{R_{41}}^{***}$
▸ EUTHYROID			
NORMAL(5)	$86 \pm 25^{*}$	22 ± 9	0.74 ± 0.07
TSH TREATED(1)	321	18	0.44
▸ GOITER			
SPORADIC (3)	670 ± 546	198 ± 182	0.83 ± 0.08
CONGENITAL(1)	1686	250	0.87
▸ HYPERTHYROID			
UNTREATED (4)	843 ± 199	280 ± 72	0.66 ± 0.02
CARBIMAZOLE TREATED (7)	1265 ± 228	390 ± 112	0.72 ± 0.04

*m $\pm$ SEM $^{**}R_{65} = \lambda_{65} \cdot V_5$ $^{***}R_{14} = \lambda_{14} \cdot V_4$

Fig. 8. Comparison of kinetic parameters of thyroid trapping estimated with ^{131}I
of Tc^{99m}. O : eythroid patients; ● : euthyroid patient after TSH stimulation;
□: hyperthyroid; ■: hyperthyroid under carbimazole; ▲: congenital goiter.

and V_5) were of the same magnitude (fig. 7A). The estimated irreversible clearance ($R_{65} = \lambda_{65} \times V_5$ averaged 22 ± 9 ml min^{-1} which is close to the accepted
value of the conventional clearance (12, 13). Furthermore the ratio R_1 of R_{14}
to R_{41} showed that 3/4 of the trapped iodide was rapidly released to plasma
(table 2).

Table 3	R_{41} (ml.min^{-1}) estimated with	
	^{99m}Tc	^{131}I
▸ EUTHYROID (3)	104	99
▸ EUTHYROID TREATED		
TSH (1)	280	320
IODINE (1)	3	25
▸ HYPERTHYROID		
UNTREATED (2)	2553	1042
TREATED (6)	986	1608
▸ CONGENITAL GOITER (1)	178	1683

With TSH stimulation, a clear increase in the thyroidal pump effectivenes:
was found (fig. 8A): enhancement of R_{41} (x 3.7) and of the iodide intrathyroid
pool $V_4 + V_5$ (x 12.5); decrease of iodide loss while the irreversible clearanc(
(R_{65}) was unmodified (table 2). These results are in agreement with what we kn(
about TSH thyroid stimulation: it is well established that the effect of TSH o1
iodide trapping and uptake are independant (14).

Sporadic and congenital goiters had the same overall picture (fig. 8B). A1
increase of the unidirectional clearance (R_{41}) was found (p<0.001); the exit r.
constants from compartment 4 or compartment 5 were decreased and the volumes V
and V_5 were much higher than these observed in the other groups (table 2). Thi:
increase means a greater amount of iodine is available for the organification
process and it is consistent with the increase of the absolute iodine uptake
previously reported (15). Furthermore, the data show two main features in the
goitrous gland: (1) 4/5 of the trapped iodide is released into plasma (2) the
irreversible clearance (R_{65}) is much higher than normal (table 2) in contrast
with normal or low serum hormonal concentration. This confirms the likelihood (
a defect in the later stages of hormone synthesis (16).

The main difference existing between euthyroid and hyperthyroid subjects
(fig. 8C) was a significant increase of R_{41} (x 10) and of the organification
rate constant λ_{65} (x 3). The two intrathyroid pools ($V_4 + V_5$) were increased
(x 11) and the irreversible clearance (R_{65}) was 13 times higher than that obse
ed in euthyroid patient. The λ_{14} loss rate constant was decreased and only 2/3
of the iodide trapped was released into the plasma.

Under antithyroid drug administration, the thyroidal undirectional cleara:

(R_{41}) was 1.5 times greater than in untreated thyrotoxic patients while the binding rate constant λ_{65} was 0.6 smaller remaining however 1.6 times above values found in euthyroid subjects. The main observation was the necessity for treated thyrotoxic patients and only for these patients, to introduce an exit rate constant λ_{16} from the bound iodine compartment 6 to the plasma. A non hormonal iodine secretion from thyroid gland has been demonstrated in euthyroid and hyperthyroid patients (17,18) but its quantity is probably too small to be detected in euthyroid patients during the 2.5 hours of the study. The perturbation imposed by carbimazole on the organic binding of radioiodide to the thyroid may enhance this non-hormonal secretion. On the other hand, the iodide release into the plasma returns to normal values.

Comparison Tc^{99m} and ^{131}I: Kinetic parameters of Tc^{99m} and ^{131}I thyroid trapping were compared in 13 patients, assuming that the binding rate constant λ_{65} for pertechnetate was non existent (19). There was a good correlation between the estimates of the total iodide and pertechnetate pools $(V_4 + V_5)$ (fig. 8A). The λ_{14} loss rate for Tc^{99m} was always higher than for iodide (fig. 8B) which is probably due to passive diffusion of pertechnetate. Table 3 shows that whereas the estimates of the undirectional clearances with TcO_4^- and ^{131}I were of the same magnitude for euthyroid patients (normal and TSH stimulated), a discrepancy exists in patients with spontaneous or acquired dyshormonogenesis.

In a case of iodine overload the decrease of the unidirectional clearance was more marked with Tc^{99m} than for ^{131}I. In two untreated thyrotoxic patients the undirectional clearance of Tc^{99m} was 2.5 higher than that estimated with ^{131}I. Under administration of antithyroid drug, undirectional TcO_4^- clearance was lower than that of iodide in the six patients studied. A similar and greater discrepancy between early ^{131}I and Tc^{99m} kinetics was observed in a patient with ongenital goiter. The technetium thyroid trap was only slightly elevated, whereas undirectional iodide clearance and $(V_4 + V_5)$ were clearly increased (fig.8).

These results underline that measurement of TcO_4^- transport may be used only as a qualitative but not quantitative index of alteration in the activity of the thyroidal iodide transport mechanism.

REFERENCES

1. Barber DC Phys. in Med. Biol. 25:283, 1980.

2. Bazin JP, Di Paola R, Gibaud P, Rougier P, Tubiana M. In: Information processing in medical imaging. Di Paola R, Kahn E (eds), Inserm, Paris, 198 p. 345.

3. DeLand FH, J. nucl. Med. 23:1, 1982.

4. Boston RC, Greif PC, Berman M, Comput. Prog. Biomed. 13:111, 1981.

5. Di Paola R, Bazin JP, Di Paola M. In: Information processing in scintigraph Metz CE, Pizer SM, Brownell GL (eds). Userda Technical Information Center, Oak Ridge, p. 115.

6. Bazin JP, Fragu P, Di Paola R, Di Paola M, Tubiana M, Eur. J. Nucl. Med. 6:317, 1981.

7. Bazin JP, Marchadier B, Lafuma J. In: Premier congrès européen de radio-protection Menton 1968, CEA Saclay, 1971, p. 374.

8. Olsson DM, J. Quality Technol. 6:53, 1974.

9. Robertson JWK, Lazarus JH, Shimmins J, Alexander WD, Horton PW. In: Dynamic studies with radioisotopes in clinical medecine and research. IAEA, Vienna, 1971, p. 199.

10. Hays MT, J. nucl. Med. 19:789, 1978.

11. Wollmann SH, Reed FE, Ann. J. Physiol. 196:113, 1959.

12. De Crombrugghe B, Beckers C, De Visscher M, Rev. Franç. Etudes Clin. et Biol. 9:307, 1964.

13. Akerman M, Di Paola R, Tubiana M, J. Clin. Endocr. Metab. 27:1309, 1967.

14. Dumont JE, Vitam. u. Horm. 29:287, 1971.

15. Tubiana M, Fragu P, De Tovar G, Bazin JP, Rev. Eur. Etudes Clin. et Biol. 16:250, 1971.

16. Tubiana M, Morvan C, Nataf BM, Ann. Endocr. Paris, 34:563, 1973.

17. Slingerland DW, Burrows BA, J. clin. Endocr. Metab. 22:368, 1962.

18. Fisher DA, Oddie T, Thompson CS, J. clin. Endocr. Metab. 33:647, 1971.

19. Fragu P, Bazin JP, Di Paola M, Tubiana M, Eur. J. Nucl. Med. 1982 (in press

THE RELATIONSHIP BETWEEN SERUM THYROGLOBULIN AND INTRATHYROIDAL
STABLE IODINE IN EUTHYROID GOITROUS PATIENTS

M.H. JONCKHEER, J. UNGER, D. COOMANS, C. DECOSTER

INTRODUCTION

The X-ray fluorescence method (XRF) enables one to estimate total stable
iodine pool (ITI) in the human thyroid gland in vivo with reasonable accuracy
and without unreasonable radiation burden (1,2). Most of the ITI is stored in
thyroglobulin (TG) (3). Higher than normal serum thyroglobulin concentrations
(sTG) have been found in various thyroid dysfunction and this has been related
to enhanced release by the thyroid cell, as a result of thyrotropin stimulation
(TSH) (4), of tissue lesion as in subacute thyroiditis or through an unknown
mechanism such as in thyroid cancer (5). The aim of the present work was to
assess whether high sTG could be related to ITI in euthyroid patients with
simple goitre.

Material and methods

97 patients were available for this study. All presented with a goitre,
but were clinically euthyroid and had basal thyroid hormones and TSH serum
concentrations within the normal range. In none circulating antithyroid antibodies (antithyroglobulin and antimicrosomes) could be detected. The ITI was
estimated by XRF (1,6) and using the functional image obtained this way, the
volume of the gland was estimated by planimetry (7). The serum concentrations
of the hormones were measured using commercially available reagents:
- thyroxine (t4) by the RIA-gnost T4 of Behringwerke (FRG); reference range
  50-110 µg/L.
- triiodothyronine (t3) by the Gamma Coat T3 RIA of Clinical Assays (USA);
  reference range 800-2000 ng/L.
- TSH by the RIA manufactured by National Institute of Radio-Elements, I.R.E.
  (Belgium); reference values between 0-7 mU/L.
- sTG following the method of Van Herle (8), reference range 120-310 µg/L.
    Intra- en interassay precision for all RIA's were within acceptable limits
(CV between 3 and 10%).

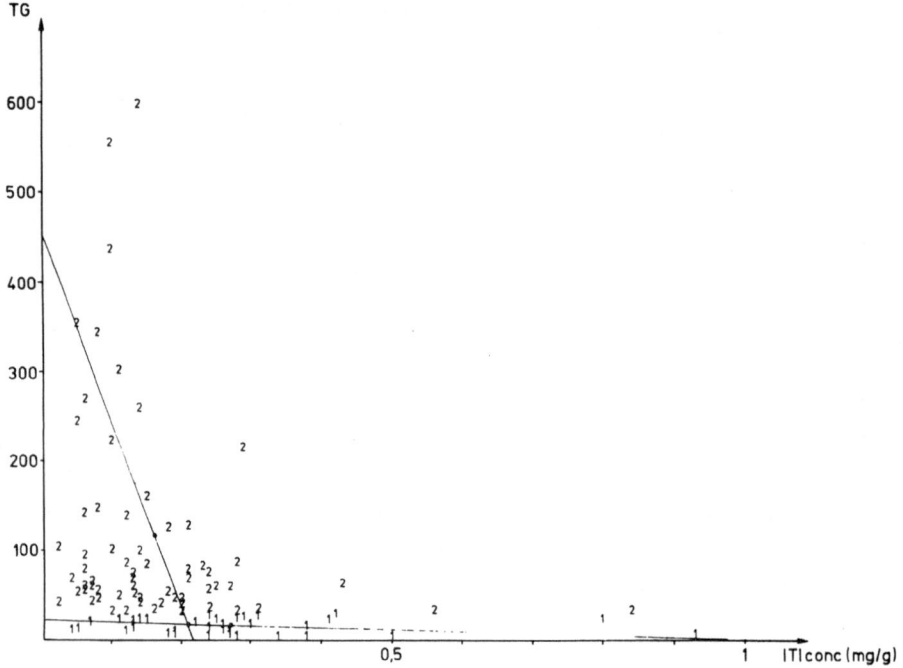

Fig. 1. Projection diagram of the patients of class 1 (1) and those of class (2) with the PC of each class after a PC multivariate analysis considering tw parameters: TG (mg/100 ml) (in ordinate) and Iconc (mg I/g tissue) (in abscis

Statistical analysis was performed after Snedecor (9) and multivariate principal components using the NIPALS procedure (10).

Results

The patients were divided into two classes: class 1 included those patie with sTG lower than 310 µg/L (upper limit of normal range) and class 2 those sTG above this limit. A principal component (PC) axis was computed for each class, using at first two parameters: sTG and intrathyroidal iodine concentra (Iconc), calculated from ITI and the volume of the gland by planimetry. The results of this analysis are represented in fig. 1. It can be seen that the class 2 patients with higher sTG values have lower Iconc values. It can also

TABLE I

PEARSON CORRELATION COEFFICIENT BETWEEN PAIRS OF PARA-
METERS CHARACTERISING THE TWO CLASSES CONSIDERED.

CLASS 1

	sTG	ITI	Iconc	Volume
ITI	0.008			
Iconc	- 0.098	0.179		
Volume	0.315	0.372	-0.086	
TSH	- 0.080	- 0.090	0.062	-0.166

CLASS 2

	sTG	ITI	Iconc	Volume
ITI	0.252			
Iconc	- 0.214	0.124		
Volume	0.283	0.161	-0.140	
TSH	0.022	0.207	0.119	-0.213

seen that there is no linear relationship between the two classes and that their
PC axes cross at an Iconc of 0.22 mgI/g tissue.

The Pearson correlation coefficients between various parameters (ITI),
Iconc, sTG, TSH and volume of the gland) were calculated. The results are represented in table I. Only significant correlations were found in both classes
between volume, ITI and sTG. No correlation could be shown between TSH and sTG,
ITI, Tconc or volume.

Another PC multivariate analysis was effectuated, using 4 parameters: ITI,
TSH, sTG and volume (adding Iconc would be redundant). In this way, the weight
coefficient of each parameter in defining the PC axis can be evaluated. The
results are represented in table II. It can be concluded that the class 1 PC is
characterized mainly by sTG and volume; ITI (accordingly Iconc) and TSH are un-
important. On the other hand, for the PX axis of class 2, sTG, ITI and volume

TABLE II

THE CONTRIBUTION OF EACH OF THE 4 PARAMETERS CONSIDERED
IN DEFINING THE PC OF BOTH CLASSES AFTER MULTIVARIATE
ANALYSIS, EXPRESSED AS WEIGHT COEFFICIENTS.

	CLASS 1	CLASS 2
sTG	+ 0.665	+ 0.459
ITI	+ 0.162	+ 0.503
VOLUME	+ 0.711	+ 0.639
TSH	− 0.160	− 0.254

are important and positively related; TSH again has a negligible weight coefficient. As the volume parameter weights more than the ITI one, it can be
concluded that sTG is negatively related to Iconc, a feature that already can b
intuitively derived by inspecting fig. 1.

Discussion

A positive correlation between sTG and TSH has been documented in endemic
goitre (11) and after intramuscular bovine TSH administration (5). Nevertheless
in a study of patients with sporadic goitre (12) 63% were found to have elevate
sTG, but no relationship could be shown between TSH concentration or size of th
glands. Our data could not relate serum TSH with sTG either. This could be due
to the poor sensitivity of the TSH RIA or to the need of a prolonged monitoring
of TSH level to detect any influence of TSH stimulation on sTG.

The alternative is of course that sTG release is triggered by a mechanism
independant from the pituitary-thyroid axis. The investigation presented here
suggests that, in that respect, one factor may be poor TG iodination, since we
found a negative correlation between Iconc and sTG. This is consistent with
findings in iodine-deficient rats (13). It is interesting to note that sTG star

to rise significantly when Iconc decreases to a level lower than 0.22 mg/g tissue: it is known that at that concentration (0.25 mg/g), as shown in vitro (14), the TG molecule undergoes spatial distortion with impairment of hormono-genesis as a result. Our studies therefore extend in vivo what had been shown in vitro. In an earlier study (15) concerning autoimmune atrophic thyroiditis, we found that the thyroid decompensates (as shown by a rise in TSH) when total ITI reaches a level lower than 2 mg I. In these studies the volume of the atrophic glands could not be estimated, but it may be assumed that their Iconc was lower than in the present investigation. These findings are therefore consist-ent and they suggest that sTG increase might be an earlier marker of thyroid insufficiency than would be the finding of an elevated TSH.

A correlation could be found between thyroid volume and sTG in both classes studied. These results are reminiscient of previous studies (16,17) but are discrepant with Pezzino's ones (12). This discrepancy could be explained by differences in methodology: although the estimation of gland size by planimetry is not very accurate (18), it certainly is more efficient than simple palpation as used by Pezzino et al. In fact, elevated sTG were to be expected in large goitrous patients either because of a mass effect or because of the presence of low iodine concentration areas in these heterogeneous thyroids (19).

Summary and conclusion

These studies demonstrate that the XRF method used clinically can yield results of physiopathological importance and confirm in vivo in man what had been implemented earlier by animal or in vitro studies. Furthermore, it allows to study thyroid disorders in basal conditions, i.e. without interference such as the administration of radioactive material or without the need of biopsy.

More specifically, they suggest the existence of a(n) (auto)regulatory mechanism of the thyroid cell whereby TG is released when Iconc reaches a level lower than 0.22 mg/g tissue.

REFERENCES

1. Hoffer PB, Jones WB, Crawford RB, Gottschalk A, Fluorescent Thyroid Scannin
   a new method of imaging the thyroid. Radiology 90:342, 1968.

2. Jonckheer MJ, Deconinck F, X-ray fluorescence determination of stable iodi
   in the thyroid gland. A review. Acta clin. belg. 1982 (In press).

3. DeGroot LJ, Stanburry JB, The thyroid and its diseases. John Wiley and Sons
   New York, 1975.

4. Unger J, Van Heuverswijn C, Decoster C, Cantraine F, Mockel J, Van Herle AJ
   Thyroglobulin and thyroid hormone release after intravenous administration
   bovine thyrotropin in man. J. clin. Endocr. Metab. 51:590, 1980.

5. Van Herle AJ, Vassart G, Dumont JE, Control of thyroglobulin synthesis and
   secretion. New. Engl. J. Med. 301:307, 1979.

6. Deconinck F, Medische toepassing van halfgeleidersdetectoren. Thesis V.U.B.
   Brussels, 1977.

7. Mandart G, Erbsman F, Estimation of thyroid weight by scintigraphy. Int. J.
   Nucl. Biol. 2:185, 1975.

8. Van Herle AJ, Uller R.P. Matthews NC, Brown J, Radioimmunoassay for measure
   ment of thyroglobulin in human serum. J. clin. Invest. 62:1320, 1973.

9. Snedecor GW, Statistical Methods, Iowa State University Press, Ames. 1956.

10. Wold H, Non linear estimation by iterative least squares procedures. In:
    Festschrift for J. David FN (ed), Weyman, Wiley, New York, 1966.

11. Ibbertson HK, Endemic goitre and cretinism. Clin. Endocr. Metab. 8:100, 197

12. Pezzino V, Vigneri R, Squatrito S, Filetti S, Camus M, Polosa P, Increased
    serum thyroglobulin levels in patients with nontoxic goitre. J. clin. Endoc
    Metab. 46:653, 1978.

13. Van Herle AJ, Klandorf H, Uller RP, A radioimmunoassay for serum rat thyro-
    globulin: physiologic and pharmacologic studies. J. clin. Invest. 56:1073,
    1975.

14. Ermans AM, Kinthaert J, Camus M, Defective intrathyroidal iodine metabolism
    in non-toxic goitre: inadequate iodination of thyroglobulin. J. clin. Endoc
    Metab. 28:1307, 1968.

15. Jonckheer MJ, Vanhaelst L, Deconinck F, Michotte Y, Atrophic autoimmune
    thyroiditis. Relationship between the clinical state and intrathyroidal iodi
    as measured in vivo in man. J. clin. Endocr. Metab. 53:476, 1981.

16. Shlossberg AH, Jacobson JC, Ibbertson HK, Serum thyroglobulin in the diagno
    and management of thyroid carcinoma. Clin. Endocr. 10:17, 1979.

17. Torrigiani J, Doniach D, Roitt IM, Serum thyroglobuline levels in healthy
    subjects and in patients with thyroid disease. J. clin. Endocr. 29:305, 196

18. Lukas WP, Leisner B, Fink U, Seiderer M, Pickardt CR, Lissner J, Sonogra-
    phische Volumebestimming der Schilddruse. Vergleich mit anderen Methoden.
    Nuklearmedizin 20:64, 1981.

19. Reutsch H, Studer H, Frauchiger B, Siebenhuner L, Topographical heterogenei
    of basal and TSH stimulated adenyl cyclase activity in human nodular goiter
    J. clin. Endocr. 53:507, 1981.

WHY DOES SOME GENERATOR-PRODUCED PERTECHNETATE-99m FAIL
TO CONCENTRATE IN THYROID?

S.K. SHUKLA, G.B. MANNI, C. CIPRIANI, G. ARGIRÒ

INTRODUCTION

The thyroid gland is one of the organs frequently imaged in nuclear medicine laboratories (1). The most commonly used radiopharmaceutical for its visualization is the pertechnetate-99m ion. During our studies over several years using the generator-produced pertechnetate-99m ion, we sometimes observed a more or less diffused concentration of Tc^{99m} in the neck of the patient with no image of the thyroid gland. Chromatographic and electrophoretic examination of this pertechnetate-99m eluate showed the anion to be transformed into other $Tc99m$ species with chromatographic and electrophoretic behaviour quite different from that of the pure pertechnetate-99m ion. The quality of the thyroid scintigram depended on the amount of the free pertechnetate-99m present in the eluate.

Since the impurity that may contaminate the pertechnetate-99m ion could be aluminum from the generator alumina column, we searched for its presence in the eluate. We had previously reported (2) that the presence of 4 µg/ml of aluminum in the eluate of 200 mCi generator is sufficient to make pertechnetate-99m anion unable to concentrate in the thyroid gland, and may even change its ionic nature. Since then quality control of the pertechnetate-99m eluate before its injection for thyroid, brain or salivary gland imaging or preparation of other Tc^{99m} radio-pharmaceuticals has become daily practice in our laboratories. We report here our further findings with pertechnetate-99m ion eluates that do not localize in the thyroid gland.

Materials and methods

Pertechnetate generators used in our laboratories are DRN 4329 Ultratechnekow FM from Byk-Mallinckrodt CIL B.V. Petten, The Netherlands; Elumatic III Tc^{99m} Sterile Generators from CIS CEA Sorin, Saluggia, Italy, or from Behring, West Germany. The chromatographic and electrophoretic procedures used have been described in detail elsewhere (2). The presence of aluminum in the pertechnetate-99m eluate was detected by aluminon spot test (3). Aluminum was determined

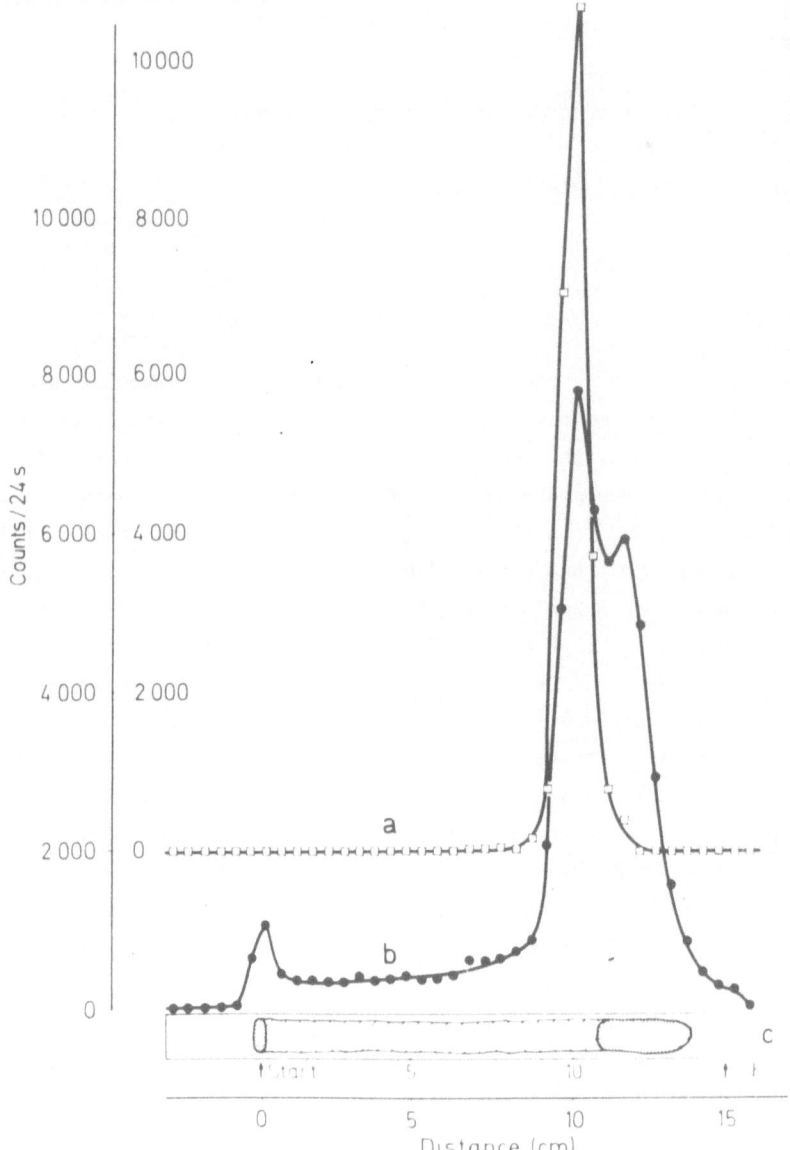

Fig. 1a. Radiochromatogram of chromatographically pure pertechnetate-99m ion
1b. Radiochromatogram of pertechnetate-99m ion eluate containing 4 μg/ml of aluminum.
1c. Chromatogram of aluminum chloride in physiological saline. Chromatograph system: physiological saline - Whatman 3 MM paper.

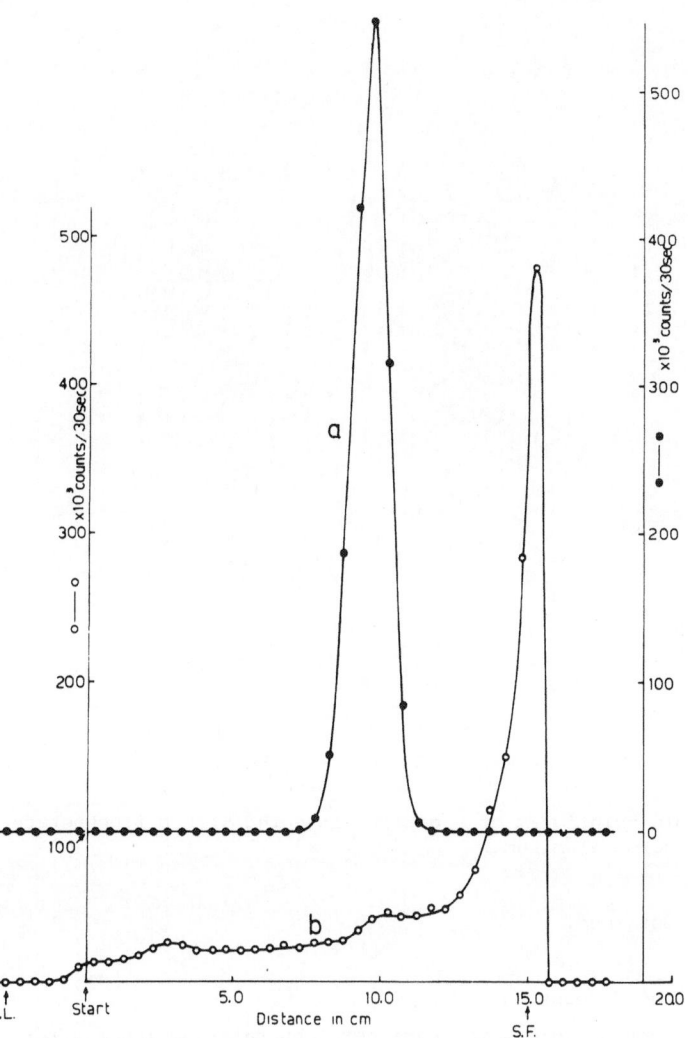

Fig. 2a. Radiochromatogram of chromatographically pure pertechnetate-99m ion.
2b. Radiochromatogram of pertechnetate-99m ion eluate containing 6 µg/ml of
aluminum.

quantitatively by Perkin Elmer Model 430 atomic absorption spectrometer connected to a model 56 recorder. The furnace tubes were of pyrolytic graphite to allow
a high number of injections be made (ca. 100). High purity argon was used to
purge the furnace at a flow rate of 900 ml/min. After decay of Tc^{99m}, the eluate
was used for the determination of aluminum. Before injection the samples were
acidified with nitric acid to 0.5 N. In physiological saline low signals for

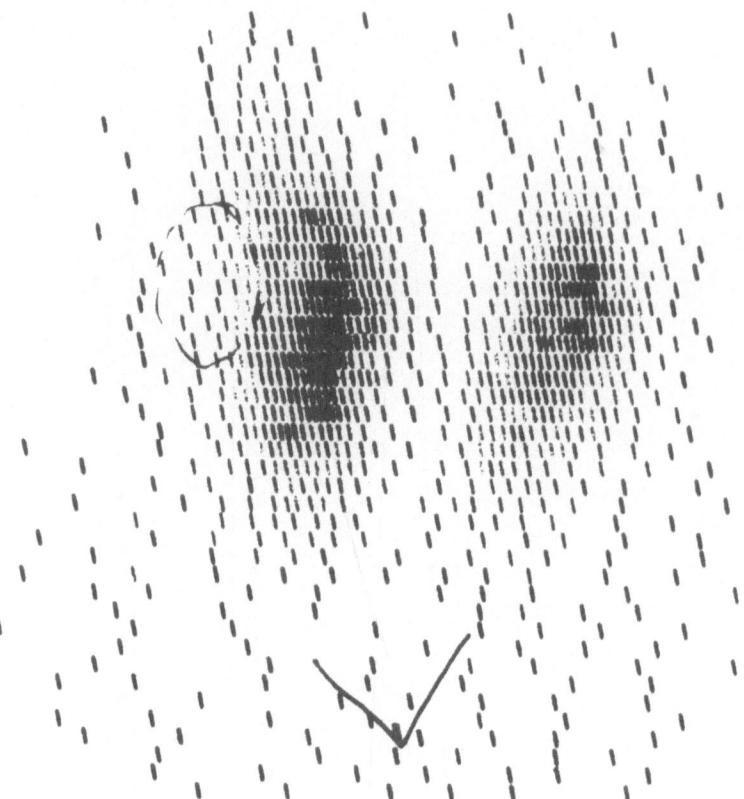

Fig. 3. Thyroid scintigram of a patient injected with pertechnetate ion elua containing 2 μg/ml aluminum.

aluminum are obtained.

Results and discussion

The radiochromatograms for pure pertechnetate-99m ion and for generator produced eluates containing 4 and 6 μg/ml aluminum are shown in figs. 1 and ? Chromatographically pure pertechnetate-99m ion has a single sharp chromatog band at R_f value of 0.65 in the chromatographic system: Whatman 3MM- physio-logical saline at room temperature. Cationic aluminum complexes (2) with per technetate-99m ion to form anionic tetra-pertechnetate-99m-aluminate (III) according to the reaction:

$$4 \ ^{99m}TcO_4 \ + \ Al^{3+} \ \rightarrow \ (Al(^{99m}TcO_4^-)_4)^-$$

Tetrapertechnetate-99m-aluminate

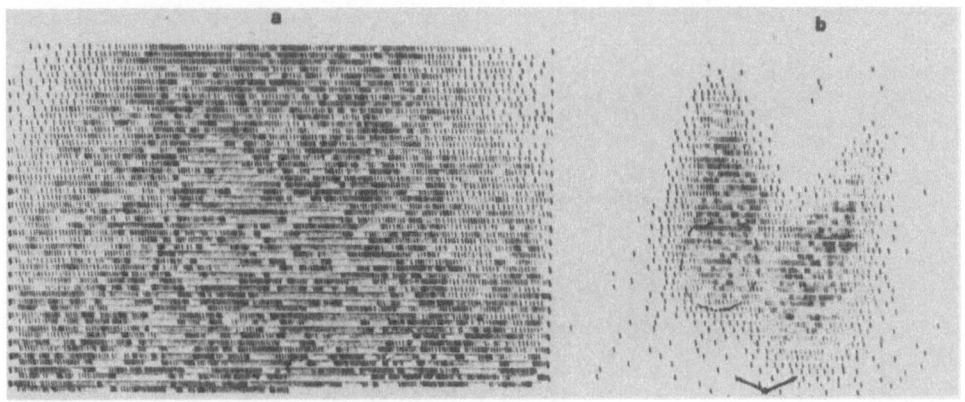

Fig. 4a. Scintigram of a patient injected with pertechnetate-99m ion eluate
containing 4 µg/ml aluminum.
4b. Scintigram of the patient of fig. 4a injected with chromatographically pure
pertechnetate-99m 24 hours later.

which is anionic in electrophoresis and also gives a sharp chromatographic band

near the solvent front (R_f = 1.00) in 200 mCi pertechnetate-99m eluate containing

6 µg/ml aluminum (fig. 2b). At lower aluminum concentrations, two bands corres-

ponding to the pertechnetate-99m ion and to the tetrapertechnetate-99m-aluminate

(III) are obtained (fig. 1b). In physiological saline tetrapertechnetate-99m-

aluminate (III) undergoes some aquation and hydrolysis to produce other anionic,

neutral and cationic pertechnetate-99m-aluminum species in electrophoresis and

many species behind the chromatographic spot of the tetrapertechnetate-99m-

aluminate (III) in the radiochromatogram (fig. 1b).

Since the thyroid gland concentrates only anionic species, such as ^{131}I and

$^{99m}TcO_4^-$, the thyroid image is not obtained by injecting generator-produced per-

technetate-99m eluate containing Al^{3+} sufficient to complex all or much of the

pertechnetate-99m ion (figs. 4a and 5a). When aluminum containing solutions of

pertechnetate-99m are aged, some free pertechnetate-99m is reproduced due to

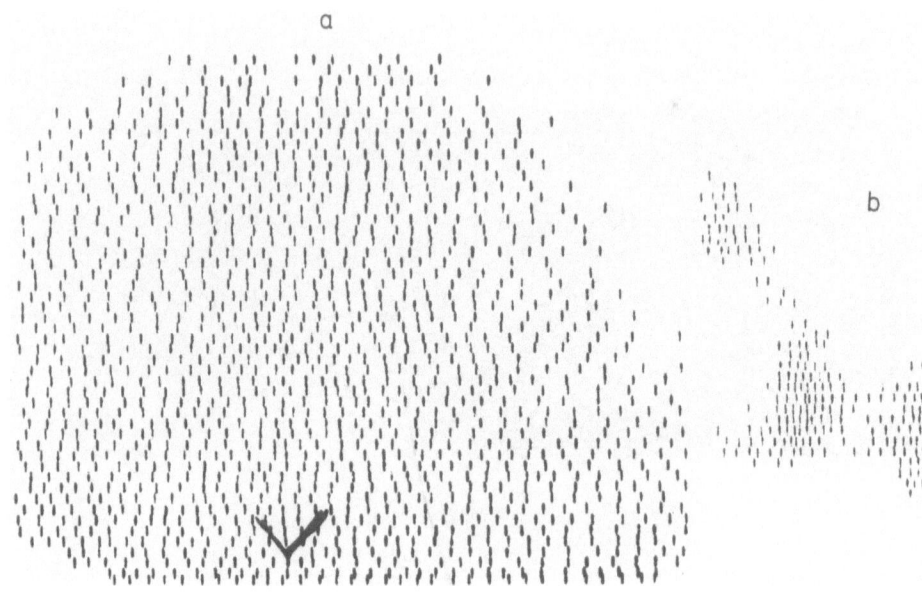

Fig. 5a. Scintigram of a patient injected with pertechnetate-99m ion eluate containing 6 µg/ml aluminum.
5b. Scintigram of the patient of fig. 5a injected with chromatographically]
pertechnetate-99m 24 hours later.

hydrolysis of the tetrapertechnetate-99m–aluminate (III). Such effects were marked in 4 µg/ml aluminum containing eluates. Figs. 3, 4a and 5a show thyr‹ scintigrams of patients injected with 2,4 and 6 µg/ml aluminum containing p‹ technetate-99m eluates. Pure pertechnetate-99m injected in the same patients high quality scintigrams (figs. 4b and 5b). These scintigrams were obtained hours following the injection of aluminum containing pertechnetate-99m elua This shows that the pertechnetate-99m–aluminum (III) species concentrated i the neck are readily eliminated and do not interfere with later imaging stu‹

Conclusion

Pure pertechnetate-99m ion gives a single sharp band at the R_f value o: 0.65 in the chromatographic system: physiological saline – Whatman 3MM pape: The presence of Tc^{99m} radioactivity at other points of the radiochromatogra: due to pertechnetate-99m–aluminate (III) (R_f = 1.00) or its hydrolysis prod:

The pertechnetate-99m-aluminate is formed in the eluate of the generator by reaction of the pertechnetate-99m ion with aluminum formed by hydrolysis of the alumina. Since only pertechnetate-99m anion concentrates in the thyroid, the aluminum modified pertechnetate-99m species, which are bulky or no longer anionic in nature, do not concentrate in this gland and one observes a diffused radio-activity distribution in the neck of the patient.

REFERENCES

1. Anonym, Evaluation of diseases of the thyroid gland with the in vivo use ⟨ radiopharmaceuticals, J. nucl. Med. 19:107, 1978.

2. Shukla SK, Manni GB, Cipriani C, Effect of aluminium Impurities in the Generator-produced pertechnetate-99m ion on thyroid scintigrams, Europ. J. Nucl. Med. 2:137, 1977.

3. Feigl F, Spot Test, Vol. I, Inorganic Applications, 4th Ed. Elsevier Sci. Publ. Co. Amsterdam, 1954, p. 181.

THE KINETICS OF THALLIUM^{201} UPTAKE IN THYROID CARCINOMA

J. TENNVALL, J. PALMER, E. CEDERQUIST, M. ÅKERMAN

INTRODUCTION

A solitary area in a thyroid scintigram which shows no evidence of uptake of iodine or technetium pertechnetate represents a carcinoma until proven other- wise. This general rule is not acceptable in the preoperative diagnosis of thyroid cancer because a cold area can be produced by several other lesions. Preoperative aspiration biopsy cytology of the thyroid is often not conclusive. The aim of this study is to assess the role of thallium scintigraphy including kinetic studies in the diagnosis of suspected thyroid cancer as a complement to conven- tional thyroid scintigraphy and preoperative aspiration biopsy cytology.

Patients and methods

Patients. In a study of 100 patients in whom the final diagnosis was established by histology, we have investigated the potential of thallium-201 in increasing the specificity of tumour detection. The criteria for inclusion in this study were an iodine- or technetium scintigram showing a solitary area with reduced or absent uptake (fig. 1). The retention kinetics were evaluated in a series of 36 patients.

Methods

Sequential imaging was performed with a pinhole-equipped scintillation camera- The kinetic data were obtained, following intravenous injection of 1-2 mCi (37-74 MBq) ^{201}-Tl-chloride, using a Pho Gamma III HP camera with digital storage on magnetic tape. Data were recorded at 2 min intervals during a period of 40 min. To identify lesions, static images with $^{99}Tc^{m}$-pertechnetate were made after the dynamic study, in the same position. The method has been improved to run as a simultaneous double-isotope study on a General Electric Portacamera IIc connected to a DEC GAMMA-11 system.

In order to eliminate errors due to the normal variations between individ- uals, due to patient positioning and callibration effects, the pathological

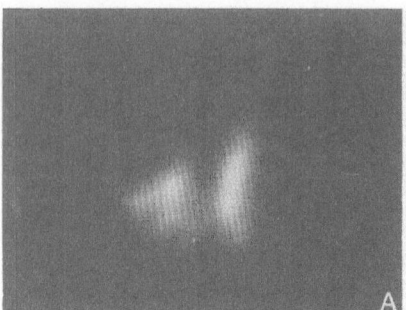

Fig. 1. A, B. Comparison between technetium- (1A) and thallium scintigram (1B) in the same patient. The technetium scintigram shows a defect in the cranial pɑ of the right lobe while the thallium scintigram shows an increased uptake on th corresponding site. The histopathology revealed a papillary carcinoma on this location.

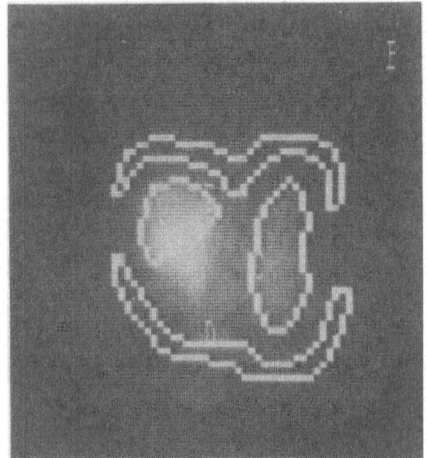

Fig. 2. Regions of interest in the thallium scintigram showing pathological, normal and background areas. The pathological region was primarily defined from the simultaneous technetium scintigram.

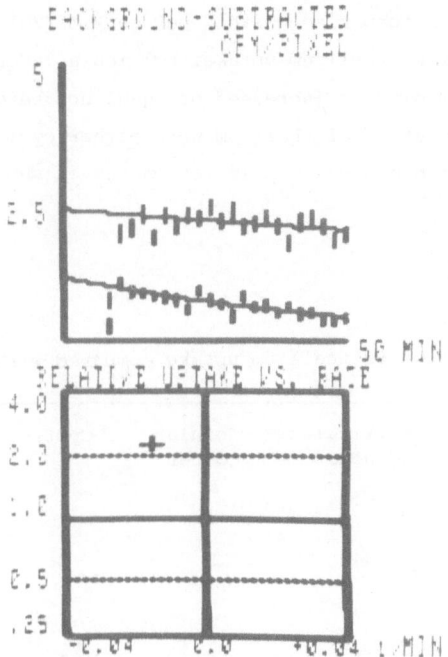

Fig. 3. Example of kinetics of thyroid thallium[201] uptake for the same patient
as in figs. 1 and 2. Top: Elimination curves in normal (below) and cancerous
tissue (above). Bottom: Diagram showing the extrapolated zero-time uptake ratio
(C_p/C_n) and relative disappearance rate ($\lambda_p - \lambda_n$). The current values are located
in the quadrant assigned to an increased uptake and delayed elimination.

region has been related to a normal region in each patient (fig. 2).

Data is thus analysed in terms of the relative uptake (C_p/C_n) and relative

elimination rate ($\lambda_p - \lambda_n$), obtained by fitting single exponential functions

(C exp(-λt)) to curves generated from normal (n) and pathological (p) regions-of-

interest, as defined primarily by $^{99}Tc^m$ (or ^{131}I) images. The count-rates are

area-normalized and backgroud-substracted, and the fits are made during the time

interval 8-40 min, although the delay may usually be shortened to 6 min without

any significant change in the results. The maximum uptake occurs after 2-4 min

post injection, giving a count-rate of the order 5-10 cpm per pixel (64x64). The

clinical presentation is shown in fig. 3.

Results

The results of morphological interpretation of the thallium uptake compared

with histopathology evaluated in 100 patients are shown in table 1. In approxim-

ately 30 per cent (20/70) of the patients with increased or equal uptake the

histopathology revealed a cancer in comparison with 7 per cent (2/30) if the
scintigram showed decreased or absent thallium uptake. Follicular adenomas of
the microfollicular type usually showed an increased or equal uptake but
follicular adenomas with no accumulation of thallium were either cystic, satur-
ed with colloid or showed signs of bleeding. Cystic lesions never showed an
accumulation of thallium.

Table 1. Morphological interpretation of thallium uptake compared with
histopathology in 100 patients

	Cancer	Askanazy	Follicular adenoma	Nodular goiter	Cysts
Increased or equal uptake	20	7	34	9	0
Decreased or absent uptake	2	2	11	6	9

Table 2. Thyroid uptake and retention kinetics. Mean ± SD

Histological diagnosis	No. of patients	Rate constant λ_p min^{-1}	Relative dissappearance rate $(\lambda_p - \lambda_n)$ min^{-1}	No. of patients*	^{e}Log uptake ratio ln (C_p/C_n)
Carcinoma	7	0.015±0.007	-0.017±0.015	5	0.240±0.43
Follicular adenoma	22	0.023±0.010	-0.005±0.011	16	0.032±0.45
Nodular goiter	7	0.025±0.008	0.00 ±0.005	4	-0.061±0.44
Normal	36	0.028±0.009			

*Grossly asymmetrical glands excluded.

Dynamic studies

An analysis of dynamic data from 36 consecutive patients with cold $^{99}Tc^m$ (or ^{131}I) lesions is shown in table 2. The raw data takes the form of overlapping, roughly Gaussian distributions, with mean and standard deviation as shown. The normal tissue showed no correlation with the diagnosis of the pathological tissue in the same patient. The rate constants for cancer and adenoma are statistically separated from the normal rate of the 5% level. The separation is enhanced by the relative disappearance rate, $(\lambda_p - \lambda_n)$. The uptake ratios are difficult to evaluate because of the unknown lobe thicknesses. The values given apply when a conservative selection is made by excluding glands where the pathological lobe has an area twice or more that of the normal lobe. One of seven cancers had an uptake ratio of less than unity.

Discussion

Evaluation of thallium scintigraphy of the thyroid has been in progress for many years in various departments. Most authors agree on the general indications and findings: improving preoperative diagnosis of "cold" areas in technetium or iodine scans, which for malignant tissue shows an accumulation of thallium. The sensitivity appears to be in the region of 90-95%, while the specificity is insufficient to allow a distinction between benign lesions and cancer (1,2,3). These conclusions are in agreement with the morphological studies we have performed (table 1).

In the present study both the morphology and the kinetics have been evaluated. Neither could adequately separate cancer from follicular adenoma. Furthermore there is a correlation between thallium uptake and thyroid enlargement, which has been described earlier by Fukuchi et al (4). It should be noted that a "warm" or "hot" spot in a static image may be caused by either, or both, of an increased uptake or delayed elimination. The latter, however, may be masked by a reduced initial uptake.

The turnover was in general decreased in pathological tissues. Cancer as a group was only distinguished statistically from benign lesions by the relative disappearance rate. A low uptake is typical for non malignant tissue. When the lesion shows accumulation of thallium and in particular if the relative half-life is long the presence of a well differantiated cancer must be considered.

REFERENCES

1. Hisada K, Clinical application of 201 Tl scintigraphy in patients with col
   thyroid nodules. Clin. nucl. Med. 3, 6:217, 1978.

2. Hisada K et al. Clinical evaluation of tumour imaging with ^{201}Tl chloride.
   Radiology 129:497, 1978.

3. Palermo F et al. [201]Tl in the scintigraphic evaluation of the "cold" thyrc
   areas. Eur. J. nucl. Med. 4:43, 1979.

4. Fukuchi M et al. Uptake of thallium in enlarged thyroid glands: concise
   communication. J. nucl. Med. 20:827, 1979.

RADIOPHARMACEUTICAL DOSIMETRY IN THE TREATMENT OF DIFFERENTIATED
THYROID CARCINOMA WITH I-131

H.R. MARCUSE, C.C. DELPRAT, C.A. HOEFNAGEL, A.P.M. JONGSMA, H. MAESSEN

INTRODUCTION

Radiotherapy plans the target to non-target ratio of absorbed radiation
energy doses in advance and can fractionate its application at will by external
beams and sealed radioactive sources. The dose commitment to a thyroidectomized
patient with functioning metastases of differentiated thyroid carcinoma after
the administration of various amounts of radioiodide, is not so easily predict-
able. In this presentation the pharmacokinetics leading to the final distribution of the radiation doses and its consequences will be discussed.

Iodine Metabolism

The complication in using radioiodide is that iodine metabolism becomes
altered in a manner which is insufficiently understood. It is impossible to
calculate, from activity, an amount of activity which will deliver a therapeutically aimed dose. In fig. 1 and its tabulated legend an example is given of a
relatively small uptake after a therapeutic dose on the right and a relatively
high uptake after a previously given small tracer dose on the left. It is a
common phenomenon in patients already therapeutically treated with radioiodine
before and in patients treated for the first time. This effect and its consequences, the need for an individual dose estimation every time a patient is
treated with radioiodine, have been reported in literature several times
(1,2,3,4). The explanation for this effect is:

Large quantities of activity, offered to the functioning tissue, do
achieve an ablative state earlier than smaller amounts do.
Increasing administered doses of radioactivity result in a lower percentage
uptake combined with a shorter biological half-life.

Extraction rate

A competition exists between remnant thyroid tissue and metastatic thyroid

scintigram   isodoses   scintigram   isodoses

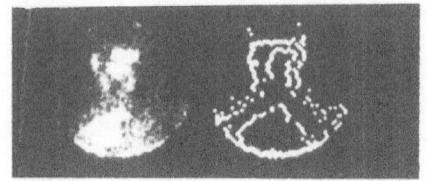 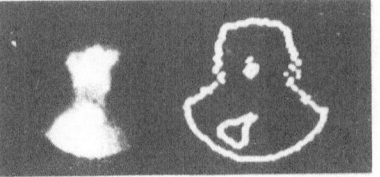

Fig.1.

Administered dose	5,68 mCi I-131 at 25-9-1978	160 mCi I-131 at 3-10-1978	in functioning metastases	
	0,04	0,01	uptake % dose	left orbita
	0,005	0,001	isodose lines	
	0,010	0,010	%D/cm²	
after 48 h	0,35	0,08	uptake % dose	right sterr
	0,005	0,001	isodose lines	clavicular
	0,010	0,010	%D/cm²	joint

head/neck   thorax/abdomen   head/neck   thorax/abdomen

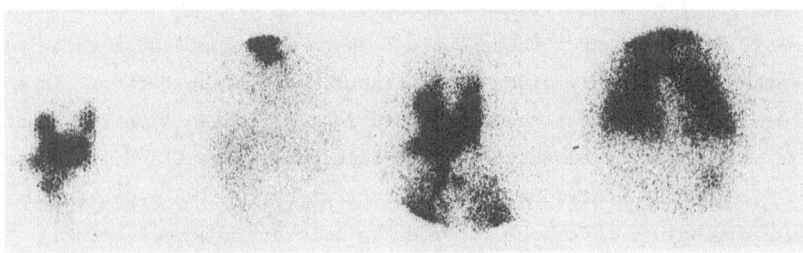

fig. 2.
96 h after: 32 mCi I-131 at 12-12-1980   197 mCi I-131 at 27-4-1981

carcinoma in the capture of the administered iodide. Fig. 2 depicts an example of follicular thyroid cancer after thyroidectomy. The situation after 96 hours is shown twice when a radioactive dose has been given: an ablative dose on the left and a subsequent therapeutic dose on the right. From fig. 3 it can be seer

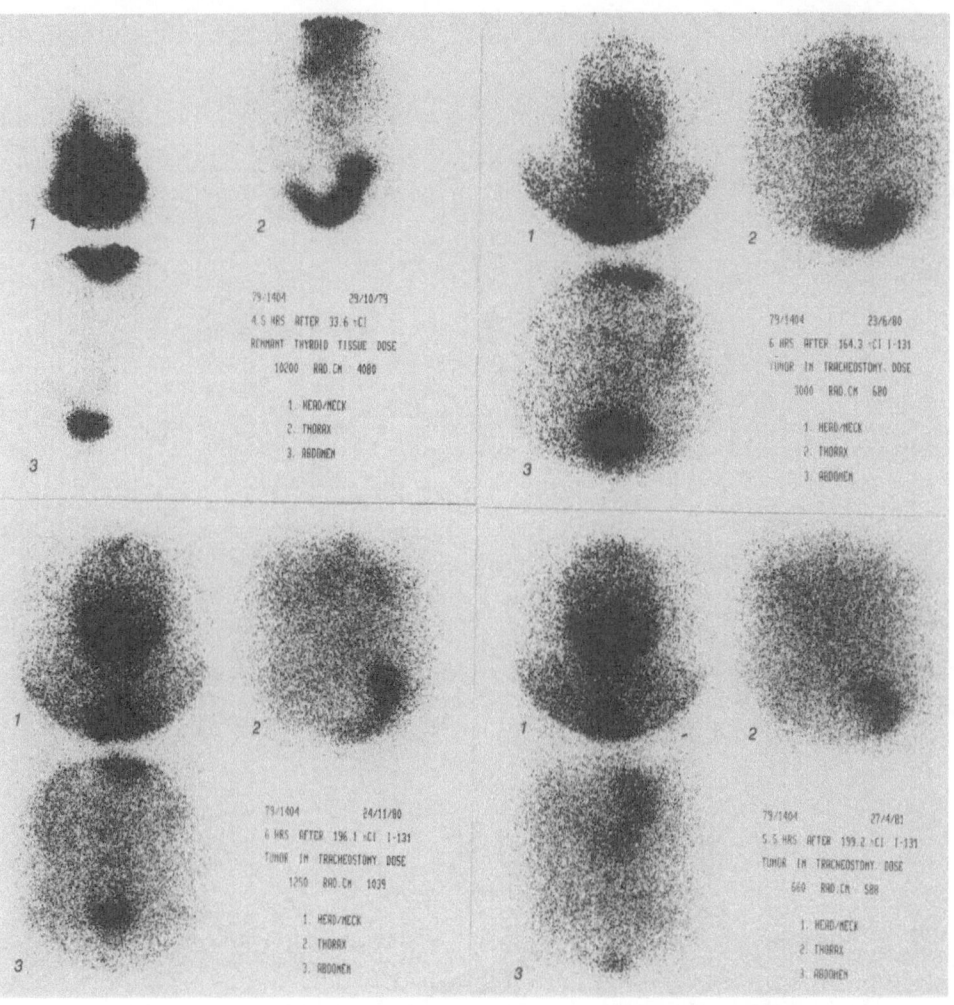

Fig. 3. The pictures can only be understood if the extraction rate of activity from plasma concentration is much greater for normal thyroid tissue than for their differentiated functioning metastases.

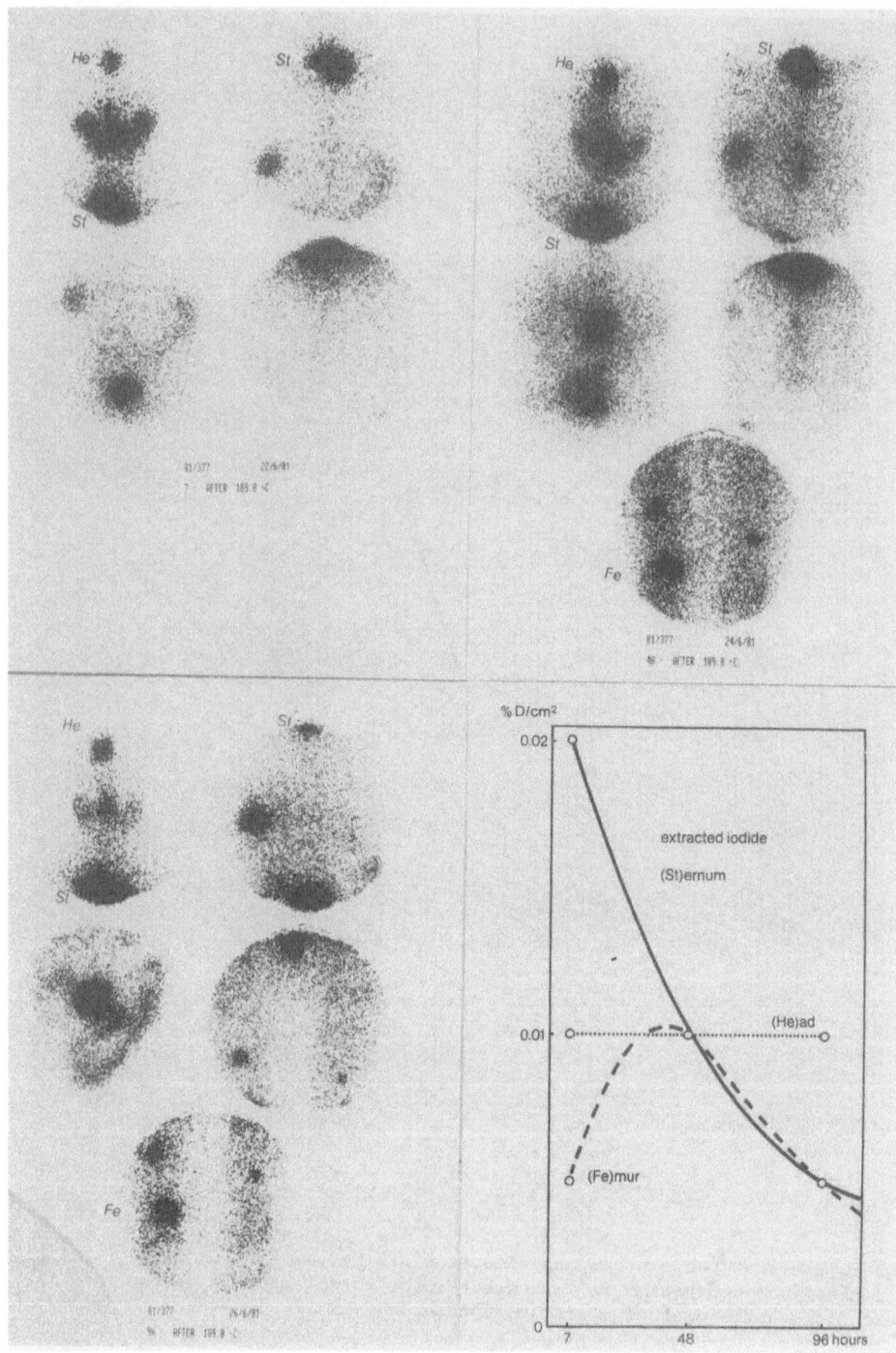

that the same tendency to visualize metastases in the absence of remnants already exists in a period much earlier, at a time when not activity can yet have been trapped by organification.

Synthesis of organic compounds

A larger fraction of the extracted activity remains in more highly differentiated thyroid carcinoma for a longer period within the synthesis of organic compounds than in poorer functioning metastasis, as shown in fig. 4. In the latter case the biological half-life may be relatively shortened.

Inhomogeneously distributed activity

The distribution of radioiodine in functional thyroid tissues occurs in clusters as has been reported earlier (5). There is evidence that this is also true for distant metastases.

Sometimes scintigraphically identified metastases have to be punctured several times, for needle biopsy under radiographic control, before radioactive cells can be removed from a lesion of a few cm³.
The geometry of the lesion, so far as for example is shown on the radiograph of fig. 5, can be known exactly. But radiographically detected beta rays from the I-131 in fig. 6 demonstrate that over a distance, that is small compared with the range of the particles, the distribution of the radioactivity in the tissue is very inhomogeneous.
Uptake in the protection of the lesion on the field of view can be measured periodically. So, the absorbed radiation dose can be calculated if the projected activity is homogeneously distributed in a layer of 1 cm thickness.
In reference (6) it has been described how this has been done by fitting so called isodose curves round the projected lesions. Dose calculations therefore, are carried out expressing the absorbed radiation dose in rad.cm, assuming the detected activity is homogeneously distributed in a tissue layer of 1 cm thickness, perpendicular to the field of view projected to the camera. Corrections have to be made for the real distribution later.

Leukemia induction dose

For the purpose of health physics each patient hospitalized for therapy with unsealed radioactive sources was monitored daily. It has been described elsewhere how these measurements were applied to estimate the radiation dose on

92

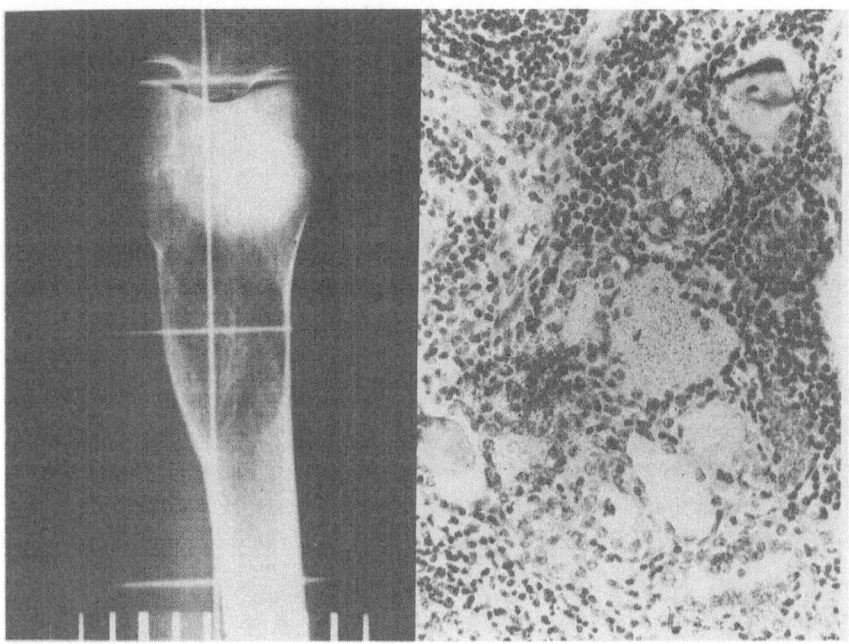

Fig. 5. 3x3x5 cm³ metastatic
lesion of follicular thyroid
ca in left femur.

Fig. 6. Tiny spikes are autoradio-
graphically detected beta rays in
the microscopic specimen emerging
from I-131 in- and outside cells
and follicles.

blood forming tissues (7). For a cumulative induction rate of 2.10^{-5} rad^{-1} th

extra probability of development of leukemia in our patients treated with I-1

is graphically shown in fig. 7. With increasing amounts of activity the extra

probability of leukemia induction was 3% per Ci I-131 administered.

Patients with thyroid remnants
in thyroid bed

Patients with thyroid tumor remnants

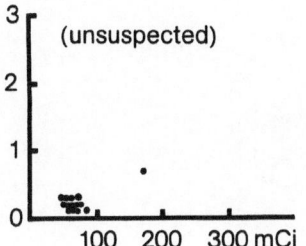

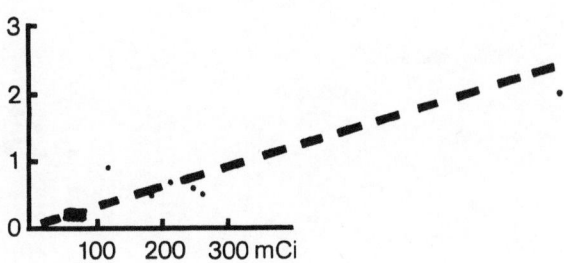

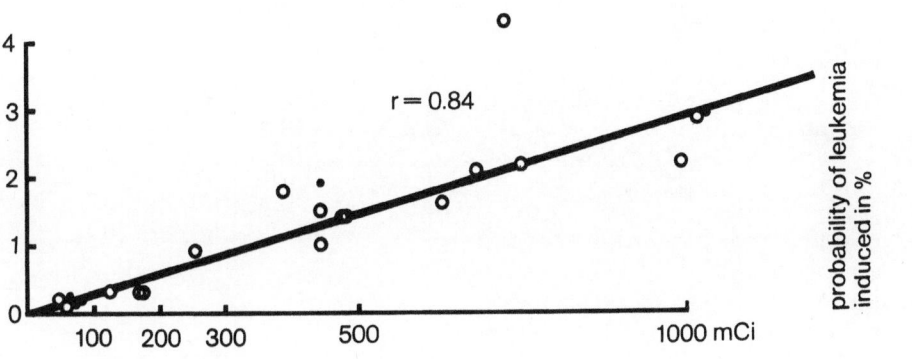

Patients with local (•) or distant (○) metastases

Fig. 7.

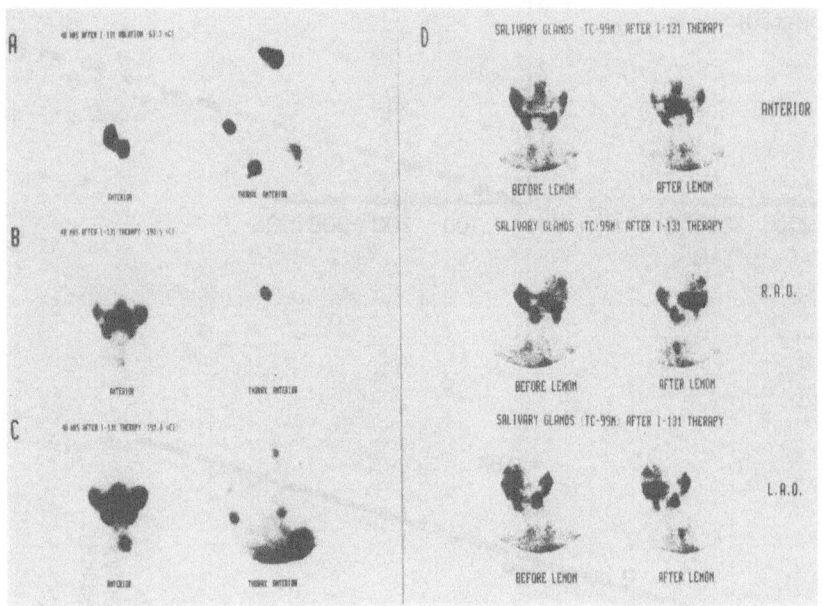

Fig. 8.

Damage to salivary glands

On total body scintigrams after therapeutic doses of I-131 .it is frequen
observed that the salivary glands concentrate a considerable amount of activi
sometime resulting in delivered doses of several hundreds of rads to these
glands. This has two aspects:

Although the salivary glands are considered to be less sensitive to rad
tion (compared with the thyroid gland) tumour induction may well occur
(8,9).

Radiation to the salivary glands can result in temporary or permanent
deterioration of the concentrative and excretory function of these gland

as is demonstrated by the following patient.

Case report

I-131 therapy was given to a 72 year old man after "total" thyroidectomy for a follicular carcinoma of the thyroid with skeletal metastases. Fig. 8 A-D.

a. 48 h after an ablative dose of 63,3 mCi of I-131 there is 4,6% dose uptake in the remnant thyroid tissue, 0,41% dose in the rib metastasis and hardly any uptake in the salivary glands.

b. Subsequent therapy with 190,5 mCi of I-131 shows total ablation of the thyroid, 0,71% dose uptake in the rib metastasis and more uptake in the salivary glands.

c. A second therapeutic dose of 191,8 mCi gives an 0,04% dose to the rib metastasis, but now a considerably higher dose to the salivary glands, especially to the left parotid gland.

d. Two months later the patient complains of a dry mouth and painful swelling of the parotid gland after meals. A salivary gland function study with 99m-Tc-pertechnetate shows decreased uptake in and excretion from the left parotid gland, suggestive of a radiation induced lesion.

Discussion

As in each patient the uptake and absorbed radiation energy dose per amount of activity administered is different, individual radiopharmaceutical dosimetry in I-131 treatment of differentiated thyroid carcinoma is necessary. The question as to how to predict the radiation doses obtained from tracer studies in thyroid carcinoma and their metastases needs further investigation. Another question is when to stop repeated therapeutic treatment with I-131 if metastatic uptake persists; is it the dosimetry that indicates the radiation dose obtained are too small, or is it that the risk of leukemia becomes too high or both? The possible harm to the salivary glands can be detected and can be prevented by correct medical intervention.

Acknowledgement

Thanks to Mr. J. Palmer of the Antoni van Leeuwenhoek Hospital for his technical assistance.

REFERENCES

1. Pochin EE, Profile counting. In: Medical Radioisotope Scanning. Seminar organized by IAEA and WHO International Atomic Energy Agency, Vienna, 195(

2. Stewart Scott J et al. Measurement of dose to thyroid carcinoma metastase: from radioiodine therapy. Brit. J. Radiol. 43:256, 1970.

3. Singh B et al. Kinetics of large therapy doses of I-131 in patients with thyroid cancer. J. nucl. Med. 15/8:674, 1974.

4. Halnan KE, The treatment of thyroid cancer. Ann. Radiol. 20/8:826, 1977.

5. Sinclair W.K. et al. A quantitative autoradiographic study of radioiodine distribution and dosage in human thyroid glands. Brit. J. Radiol. 31:36, 1956.

6. Marcuse H.R. et al. Is a comparison of I-131 treatment results by the deli ed radiation dose practicable? In: Third International Radiopharmaceutica. Dosimetry Symposium. Watson EE et al. (eds), FDA 81-8166, US Dept. of Hea and Human Services. 595-601.

7. Delprat CC et al. Retrospective blood radiation dose estimation following therapy with I-131 in thyroid carcinoma. In: Advances in Thyroid Neoplasi. Andreoli M et al. (ed), Field Educational Italy, 1981.

8. Palmer JA et al, Irradiation as an etiologic factor in tumours of the thyr parathyroid and salivary glands. Can. J. Surg. 23/1:39, 1980.

9. Stephen et al F, Irradiation induced salivary gland neoplasia, Ann. Surg. 191-304, 1980.

RADIOHALOGENATED L-α-METHYLTYROSINES AS POTENTIAL PANCREAS IMAGING
AGENTS FOR PECT AND SPECT

G. KLOSTER, H.H. COENEN, Z. SZABO, F. RITZL, G. STÖCKLIN

INTRODUCTION

The diagnosis of pancreatic carcinoma is still a problem in nuclear
medicine (1), and an improved pancreas imaging agent is urgently needed. Currently, L-I^{75}Se)-seleno-methionine (SM) is used as an agent for the detection of
pancreatic carcinoma (2), with ^{99m}Tc sulfur colloid often injected in addition
in order to permit the substraction of the interfering liver back-ground from
SM (3). This imaging procedure results in rather large radiation doses to the
patient, especially since the biological half-time of SM (70 days) is comparable
with the physical half-life (120 days) of ^{75}Se (4). Additionally, significant
numbers of false-positives and false-negatives make routine diagnosis difficult
(5).

Several attempts have been made to find suitably labelled amino acid derivatives which would accumulate in the pancreas, an organ containing preferential-
ly protein producing cells (6-13). Some of them show reasonably good pancreatic
accumulation and a useful pancreas-to-liver ratio, such as DL-(^{18}F)-phenylalanine
(6), DL-(^{11}C)-phenylglycine (9), DL-(^{11}C)-phenylalanine (9), DL-(^{11}C)-tryptophane
(10), DL-(^{11}C-valine (12) and L-(^{11}C)-methionine (13) (see table 1). Of these,
only DL-(^{11}C)-tryptophane, DL-(^{11}C)-valine (15,16) and L-(^{11}C)-methionine (14)
have found a clinical application up to now.

The fact that ^{14}C-labelled α-methyl-DOPA accumulates in pancreatic tissue
(17,18) led us to investigate its structural analogues L-3-(^{123}I)-iodo-α-methyl-
tyrosine (IMT) (19) and L-3-(^{75}Br-bromo-α-methyltyrosine (BMT) (20) as potential pancreatic imaging agents. Compared with the ^{11}C-compounds mentioned above
they have the following advantages: a) both the positron emitter ^{75}Br ($T_{\frac{1}{2}}$= 98 min)
and the single photon emitter ^{123}I ($T_{\frac{1}{2}}$= 13 h) have suitable half-lives for
clinical studies, b) easy methods for synthetizing large amounts of IMT of BMT
from the corresponding halide ions are available, and c) IMT can be used with
single photon emission computed tomography (SPECT) in institutions not having

Table 1. Radioactivity content in different organs after i.v. injection of radiopharmaceuticals, relative to radioactivity concentration in liver

L-(^{75}Se)-selenomethionine (mean of 5 animals)

	3 min	10 min	30 min	60 min
liver	18.00	17.81	17.52	17.21
	tissue to liver concentration ratio	% dose / g		
pancreas	3.32	3.47	3.43	3.06
stomach*	0.27	0.21	0.25	0.14
intestine*	0.24	0.36	0.21	0.17
spleen	0.35	0.32	0.21	0.33
kidneys	0.58	0.49	0.47	0.51

L-3-(^{123}I)iodo-α-methyltyrosine (mean of 10 animals)

	3 min	10 min	30 min	60 min
liver	7.88 ± 1.98	6.71 ± 1.88	3.03 ± 1.21	0.72 ± 0.21
	tissue to liver concentration ratio	% dose / g		
pancreas	8.38 ± 3.12	8.75 ± 1.84	9.01 ± 2.33	8.38 ± 3.67
stomach*	0.45 ± 0.20	0.41 ± 0.12	1.38 ± 0.84	2.07 ± 1.04
intestine*	0.68 ± 0.15	0.64 ± 0.10	0.94 ± 0.44	0.82 ± 0.25
spleen	1.06 ± 0.51	1.11 ± 0.36	0.82 ± 0.54	1.21 ± 0.57
kidneys	12.82 ± 2.66	16.52 ± 3.36	17.82 ± 9.06	23.11 ± 4.25

L-3-(^{75}Br)bromo-α-methyltyrosine (mean of 5 animals)

	3 min	10 min	30 min	60 min
liver	3.60 ± 0.39	1.66 ± 0.12	1.94 ± 0.12	1.30 ± 0.03
	tissue to liver concentration ratio	% dose / g		
pancreas	10.98 ± 2.93	10.53 ± 2.25	7.73 ± 1.83	9.68 ± 1.94
stomach*	1.16 ± 0.80	0.71 ± 0.18	0.72 ± 0.26	0.84 ± 0.17
intestine*	1.03 ± 0.12	0.90 ± 0.27	0.78 ± 0.11	1.02 ± 0.08
spleen	1.24 ± 0.29	1.41 ± 0.35	0.72 ± 0.17	0.76 ± 0.33
kidneys	12.63 ± 3.05	20.75 ± 6.91	21.78 ± 2.13	19.90 ± 8.59

*including contents

Table 2. Comparison of several amino acids investigated as potential pancreas-imaging agents; 30 min after i.v. injection in rats or mice

amino acid	pancreas	pancreas-to-liver ratio	animal	ref.
	% dose/organ			
DL-phenylalanine (C-11)	8.5	5.2	rat	9
DL-o-fluorophenyl-alaline (F-18)	3.0	5.2	rat	6
DL-phenylglycine (C-11)	2.2	7.0	rat	9
DL-valine (C-11)	~5	8.7	rat	12
DL-6-fluorotryptophane (F-18)	8.7	9.1	rat	7
DL-tryptophane (C-11)	-	11.0	rat	10
L-methionine (C-11)	-	2.5	mouse	13
L-3-iodo-α-methyltyrosine (I-123)	4.1	8.6	mouse	19
L-3-bromo-α-methyltyrosine (Br-75)	2.3	9.7	mouse	20
L-selenomethionine (Se-75)	9.1	3.8	mouse	19

a cyclotron and positron emission computed tomography (PECT).

In this respect the animal biodistribution data for IMT and BMT and a pr
liminary patient study using IMT will be presented.

Radiopharmaceuticals (fig. 1)

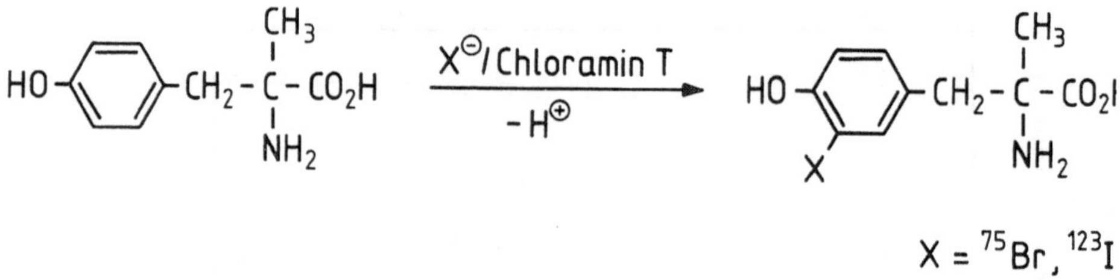

$$HO-\langle \rangle-CH_2-\underset{\underset{NH_2}{|}}{\overset{\overset{CH_3}{|}}{C}}-CO_2H \quad \xrightarrow[-H^{\oplus}]{X^{\ominus}/Chloramin\ T} \quad HO-\langle \rangle-CH_2-\underset{\underset{NH_2}{|}}{\overset{\overset{CH_3}{|}}{C}}-CO_2I$$

$$X = {}^{75}Br, {}^{123}I$$

Fig. 1. BMT and IMT are prepared from L-α-methyltyrosine by electrophilic hal
genation using halide ions (^{75}Br or ^{123}I) and an appropriate oxidizing agent
such as 10_3^- (19,21,22 or chloramine-T (22,23).

After hplc-separation of either IMT (19) or BMT (20) from the respective
halide ion and L-α-methyltyrosine, IMT was isolated in yields of 65-70% and B
with yields of 85% under no carrier added conditions. The preparation times,
cluding hplc, are less than 2 hours.

BIODISTRIBUTION IN MICE

Following i.v. administration into female NMRI mice, both IMT and BMT ar
rapidly accumulated in the pancreas (table 2) (19). Since for pancreatic imag
the relative concentration of radioactivity in the pancreas, compared with ne
organs, is more important than the absolute amount of radioactivity accumulat
(5), the data for SM, IMT and BMT are given as multiples of the liver concent
tion (cpm/g), the liver being the main interfering organ during pancreatic
imaging. During the first hour, the uptake into the pancreas is 8.6 ± 2.7 tim
as high (for IMT) and 9.7 ± 1.4 times as high (for BMT) as into the liver,
whereas the corresponding factor for SM is only 3 - 3.5. These ratios are
constant during the first 60 min within experimental error. All other organs
vestigated, except the stomach and the kidneys, exhibit rather low relative
concentrations with either IMT or BMT. The stomach concentration, which after

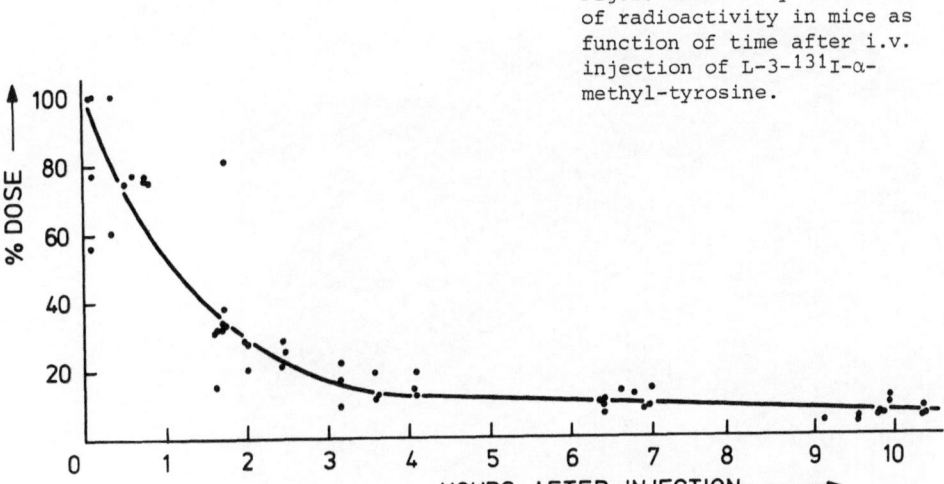

Fig.2. Whole body retention of radioactivity in mice as function of time after i.v. injection of L-3-^{131}I-α-methyl-tyrosine.

Time activity curves registered over different ROI-s of the epigastrium.

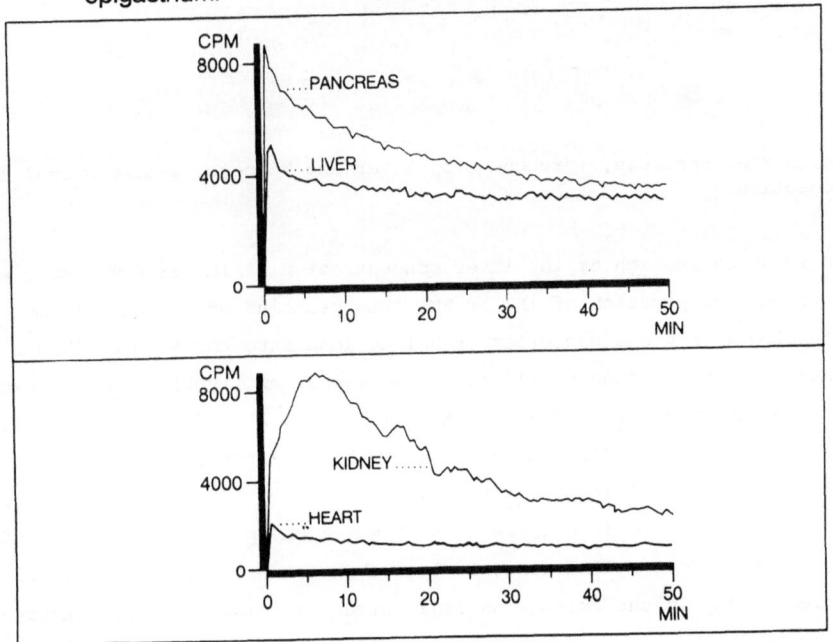

Fig. 3.

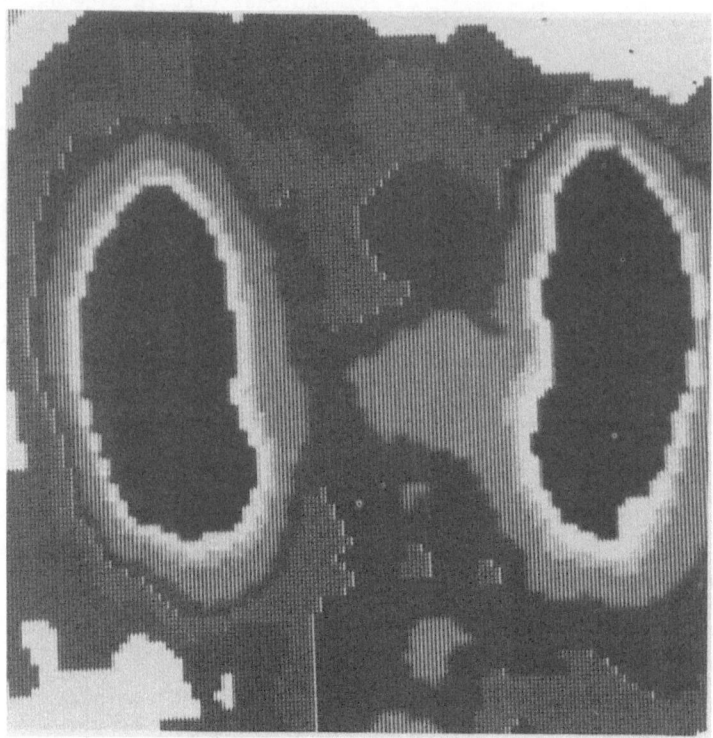

Fig. 4. Normal pancreas, surrounded by liver and kidneys, 2-dimensional in AP projection.

60 min is about as high as the liver concentration of IMT or BMT, could eith result from incorporation of IMT or BMT into proteins of the gastric mucosa from dehalogenation and excretion of halide ions into the stomach. The high concentration in the kidneys (10 to 20 times that of liver) seems to result from rapid excretion of radioactive material (fig. 2). 50% of the activity i eliminated after IMT injection in 90 min. 7 hours after administration less 10% of the dose is retained in the body.

The concentration in adipose tissue, which may provide a significant ba ground during pancreatic imaging, is less than that of the liver. Concentrat of radioactivity in the spleen, an organ directly adjacent to the pancreas, the same as in the liver, so that splenic interference should be neglegible. The thyroid contains less than 0.4% of the dose 1 hour after administration IMT; thus deiodination can only be a minor pathway in IMT metabolism.

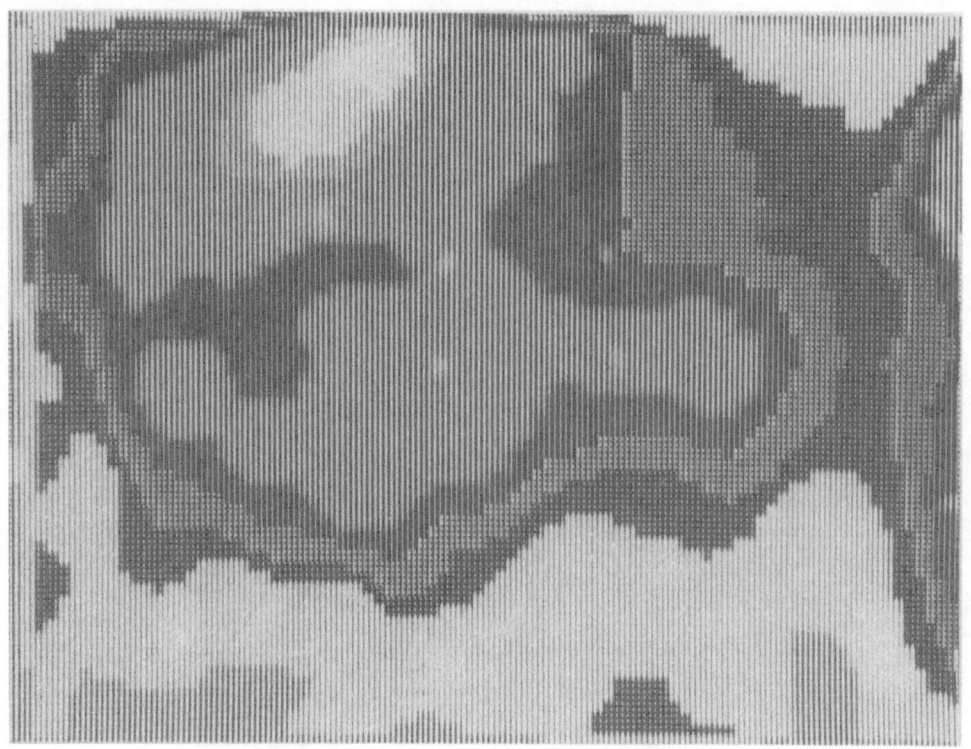

Fig. 5. Normal pancreas using seven pinhole tomography in patient with renal insufficiency.

Investigations in patients

After oral premedication with 800 mg perchlorate, sequential scintigraphy of the epigastrial areas was performed immediately after the i.v. injection of 4-10 mCi IMT. In most patients, a large field of view gamma camera was used for two-dimensional imaging, whereas in a few patients seven pinhole tomography was used in order to eliminate interfering radiation from uptake of IMT in kidney and liver.

Time activity curves (fig. 3) show an instantaneous accumulation of activity in pancreas and liver; a few minutes later, significant amounts of activity are accumulated in the kidneys. Thus, two dimensional imaging of the pancreas is difficult because of kidney interference. From sequential scintigraphy, the half-time of renal elimination was estimated to be around 55 min. Again, radiation doses are expected to be low due to this rapid excretion.

Let us consider a few selected cases to demonstrate the potential of IMT in

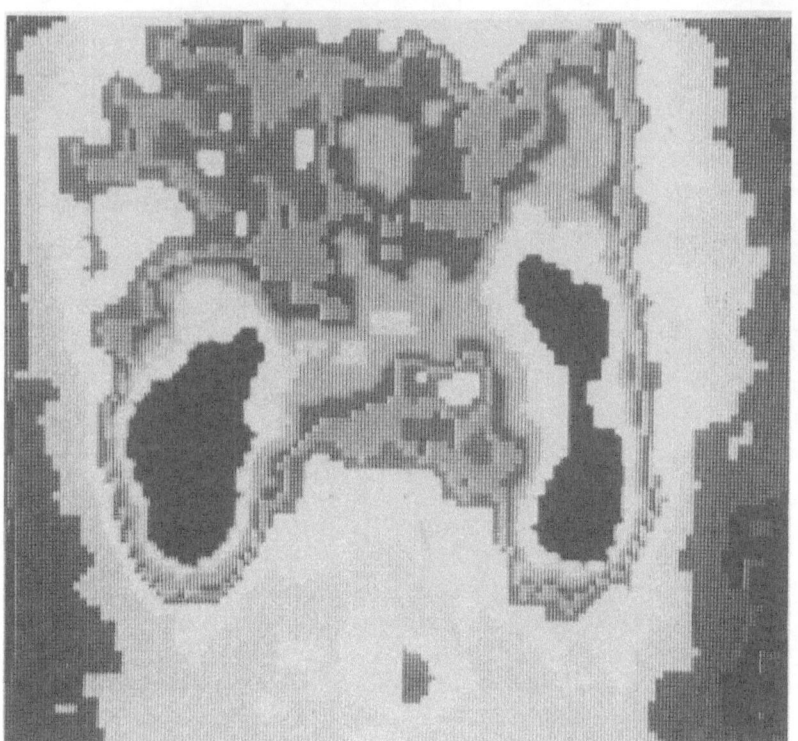

Fig. 6. Pancreatic tumour, 2-dimensional image in AP projection
(confer to fig. 3).

pancreatic imaging (figs. 4-6). Fig. 4 shows the two-dimensional image of a
normal person taken in AP projection. The body of the pancreas is clearly
visible between the kidneys. Fig. 5 shows a normal pancreas with a seven pin
hole collimator. This patient had renal insufficiency; thus, the total pancre
is clearly visible. Fig. 6. shows a two-dimensional image obtained in a patie
with carcinoma in the body of the pancreas. The activity defect in the tumour
region is clearly visible (compare to fig. 4. Fig. 7 shows a two-dimensional
image of a patient with pseudocyst of the pancreas. The cyst is clearly visib
as an activity defect within the surrounding parenchyma of the pancreas.

Discussion

To date, we have only tested IMT in patients. Since we had no access to
SPECT, the data presented here show mainly the disadvantage of IMT, namely, t
the accumulation of activity in the kidneys severely interferes with imaging

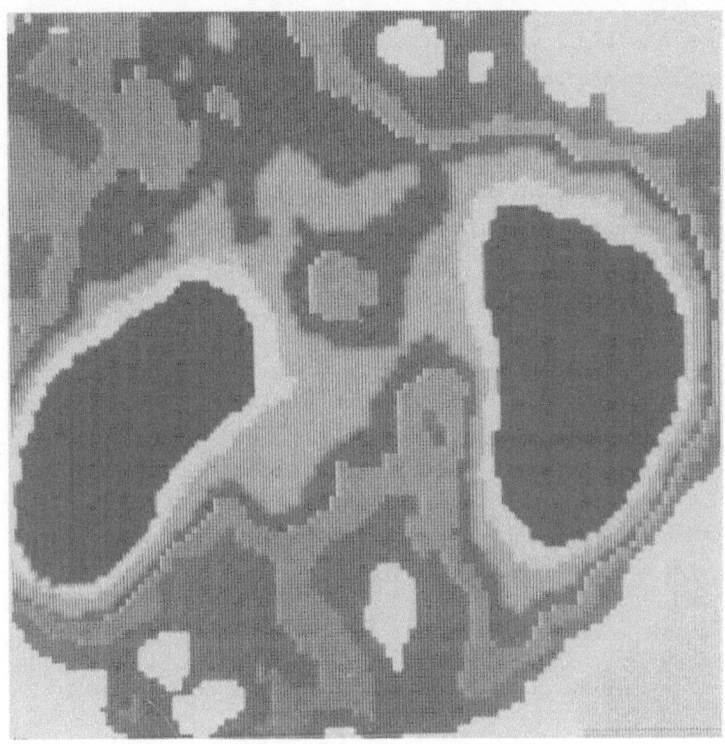

Fig. 7. Pseudocyst of the pancreas, 2-dimensional image
in AP projection (confer to fig. 3).

the head and tail of the pancreas. An obvious solution to this problem would be
the use of tomography. Seven pinhole tomography poses severe positioning
problems; only in fortunate cases, such as the one shown in fig. 5 are good
images obtained. Nevertheless, it is to be expected that useful images will be
obtained using a rotating gamma camera or similar SPECT devices.

A further possibility is the use of BMT for pancreatic imaging in conjunction with PECT. We are presently exploring this possibility. We expect that in
this case the activity accumulation in the kidneys should not be a problem. This
can be seen in the case of L-(^{11}C)-methionine (14), DL-(^{11}C)-valine and DL-(^{11}C)
tryptophane(15,16), where no kidney interference was noted, even though kidney
activity accumulation was significant.

Compared to these ^{11}C-labelled amino acids, IMT and BMT have the following
advantages: a) both the positron emitter ^{75}Br ($T_{\frac{1}{2}}$ = 98 min) and the single
photon emitter ^{123}I ($T_{\frac{1}{2}}$ = 13 h) have more suitable half-lives for clinical

studies than ^{11}C ($T_{\frac{1}{2}}$ = 20.3 min); b) efficient methods for synthetisizing la
amounts of IMT and BMT from the corresponding halide ions are available; and
c) IMT in conjunction with SPECT offers an alternative to SM for institution
not having a cyclotron and PECT.

In conclusion, we feel that IMT and BMT are pancreas imaging agents whi
deserve further clinical studies in conjunction with either SPECT or PECT.

REFERENCES

1. McAfee JG. In: Radiopharmaceuticals. The Society of Nuclear Medicine, Subramanian G, Rhodes BA, Cooper JF et al. (eds), New York, 3:14, 1975.

2. Blau M, Manske RF, J. nucl. Med. 2:102, 1961.

3. Zurowski S, Graban WT, Jabukowski W, Eur. J. nucl. Med. 2:273, 1977.

4. Lathrop KA, Johnston RE, Blau M, Rothschild EO, J. Nucl. Med. 13, suppl. 6:7, 1972.

5. Quinn JL, III. In: Nuclear Medicine, Wagner HN, jr, (ed), HP Publising Comp. New York, 153-160, 1975.

6. Hoyte RM, Lin SS, Christman DR, Atkins HL, Hauser W, Wolf AP, J. nucl. Med. 12:280, 1971.

7. Atkins HL, Christman DR, Fowler JS, Hauser W, Hoyte RM, Klopper JF, Lin SS, Wolf AP, J. nucl. Med. 13:713, 1972.

8. Lambrecht RM, Atkins H, Elias H, Fowler JS, Lin SS, Wolf AP, J. nucl. Med. 15:863, 1974.

9. Vaalburg W, Beerling- van der Molen HD, Woldring MG, Nucl. Med. 14:60, 1975.

10. Washburn LC, Wieland BW, Sun TT, Hayes RL, Butler TA, J. nucl. Med. 19:77, 1978.

11. Kung HF, Gilani S, Blau M, J. nucl. Med. 19:393, 1978.

12. Washburn LC, Sun TT, Byrd BL, Hayes RL, Butler TA, J. nucl. Med. 20:857, 1979.

13. Comar D, Cartron JC, Mazière M, et al. Eur. J. nucl. Med. 1:11, 1976.

14. Syrota A, Comar D, Cerf M, Plummer D, Mazière M, Kellershohn C, J. nucl. Med. 20:778, 1979.

15. Buonocore E, Hübner KF, Radiology 133:195, 1979.

16. Hübner KF, Andrews GA, Buonocore E, Hayes RL, Washburn LC, Collmann IR, Gibbs WD, J. nucl. Med. 20:507, 1979.

17. Duhm B, Maul W, Medenwald H, Patzschke K, Wegner LA, Z. Naturforschg. 20b:434, 1965.

18. Duhm B, Maul W, Medenwald H, Patzschke K, Wegner LA, Schlossmann K, Z. Naturforschg, 22b:70, 1967.

19. Tisljar U, Kloster G, Ritzl F, Stöcklin G, J. nucl. Med, 20:973, 1979.

20. Ritzl F, Kloster G, Coenen HH, Tisljar U, Stöcklin G, J. nucl. Med. 22:87, 1981, (abstract).

21. Kloss G, Becker H, Niemann E, Leven M, Patent 21,45,282 (Fed. Rep. Germany) 1975.

22. Kloss G, Leven M, Eur. J. nucl. Med. 4:179, 1979.

23. Petzold G, Coenen HH, J. Lab. comp. Radiopharm. 18:1319, 1981.

STEROID METABOLISM IN THE ADRENAL CORTEX

J. FRÜHLING

INTRODUCTION

Isotopic investigations using ^{131}I- or ^{75}Se-labelled cholesterol constitute an interesting technique for the in vivo diagnosis of morphological or functional disorders of the human adrenal cortex. The aim of this short review paper is to present the essential part of ultrastructural morphological and biochemical data allowing the true interpretation of results obtained by means of the scintigraphic or functional isotopic investigations. This article constitutes in fact an extended summary of the last and most up to date review articles existing in the literature (1-5), and of the authors own thesis (6), devoted to the same subject.

Materials and methods

Studies of the correlation between morphology and function, especially at the ultrastructural level are a particular problem. The greatest part of the classical investigation methods in the field of molecular biology has been adapted to the study of steroid metabolism in the adrenal cortex. These modifications, due to the high lipid content of the gland and of the subcellular components, concern the scheme of ultra-centrifugation, the cytochemical techniques and several steps in the fixation, dehydration and embedding of the tissue during the preparation for ultrastructural morphological studies. The specificity of these modifications and the rational use of the combined morphological (descriptive and morphometric, cytochemical, autoradiographic, biochemical and radiochemical analysis of the whole adrenal cortex and of the isolated subcellular fractions is described in detail in the thesis cited above (6).

Contributions

I. Generalities. The adrenal cortex, the most complex and the most thoroughly studied of the steroid secreting endocrine glands is constituted of at least three distinct zones characterized by specific cytological features of the cells and by their arrangement. This tripartite zonation is most clearly demonstrable

in adrenals, containing an important amount of lipid droplets (man, monkey, r
mouse, guinea-pig, etc). In the lipid-poor adrenals (cow, horse, etc.) the di
tinction between the zones is less clear. According to well accepted experime
results these morphological unities should correspond to regions with specifi
metabolic tasks. Thus, the exterior, so called, zona glomerulosa products the
salt-regulating hormone aldosterone, while the interior zones - fasciculata a
reticularis - secrete (depending upon the species) glucocorticoids and androg
under the controle of the pituitary ACTH. Among these zones the inner one, th
reticularis should be the site of androgenic steroid secretion, but the evide
of this last mechanism remains yet contradictory.

In some species, such as the rat, there is a fourth, intermediate or sudi
phobic zone, situated between the glomerulosa and the fasciculata, correspond
to the site of the cell division and the organ regeneration.

II. Ultrastructural morphology

(The material discussed in this and in the following sections mainly
concerns the rat, which belongs nevertheless to the same group of species, wi
high lipid and steroid content, as the man).

On the electromicroscopical level the different layers can be distinguis
according to the morphology of their mitochondria and to the intracellular vo:
occupied by the different subcellular organites, as established by the morpho
metric analysis. Thus, the zona glomerulosa is containing mitochondria with
abundant matrix and short tubular cristae, some of them presenting a paracris
talline organization. The zona fasciculata presents mitochondria where the
greatest part of the mitochondrial volume is occupied by the tubulosaccular
cristae. The external fasciculata contains a high amount of lipid droplets
(12,9% of the total cell volume) whereas in the internal fasciculata the volu
occupied by the liposomes falls to 4,1%; the smooth endoplasmic reticulum (ER
representing the most aboundant (± 50% of cell volume) intracellular organite
In the zona reticularis the mitochondria are greater, present more matrix and
a lesser amount of cristae, which are larger and mostly saccular. The smooth
ER is the best developed in this zona. A constant amount of the mitochondria
the inner zones present groups of round lipid inclusions with a diameter of 3
to 120 nm. The smooth and rough ER constitute in all zones a morphological
entity composed by a network of tubular elements with a diameter varying betw
35 and 75 nm. (For all details: see fig. 1).

Cytochemically digitonine present in the aldehydic fixative allows the

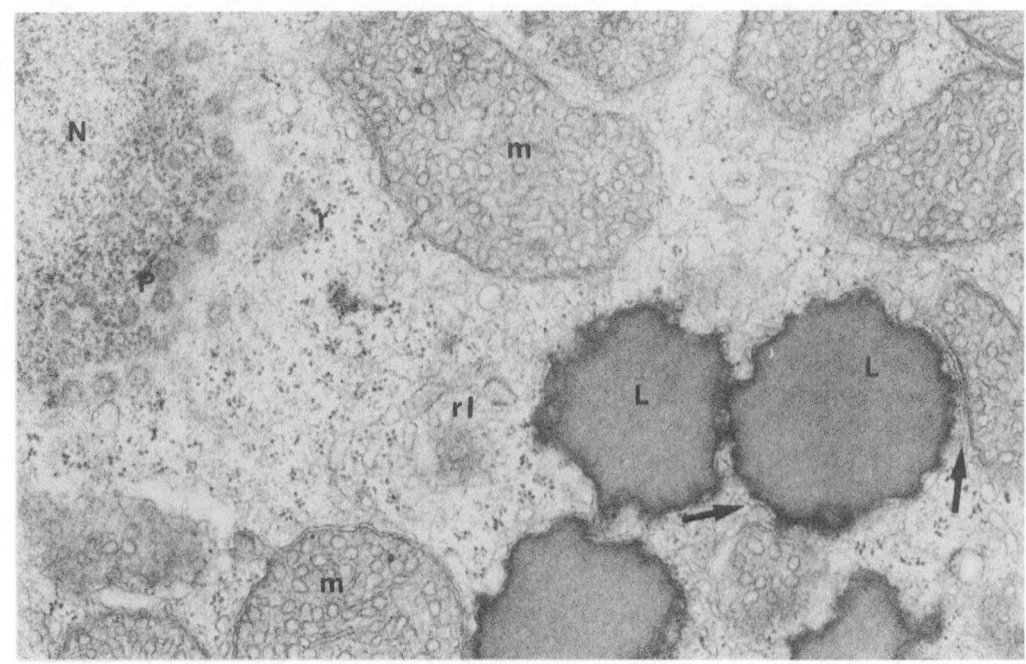

Fig. 1. Rat adrenal cortex: external fasciculata zone; cell detail. N : nucleus
with tangential sections of nuclear pores (P). m : mitochondria filled with
tubulosaccular cristae. rl : network of smooth endoplasmic reticulum. r: free
ribosomes and polysomes. L : lipid droplets in close contact (arrows) with the
elements of endoplasmic reticulum and with mitochondria.
Fixative: OsO_4 4% in bidistilled water; dehydratation with 70% ethanol as
highest liposolvent concentration used; "Epon 812" embedding. Contrasted by
uranyl-acetate and lead-citrate. x 30 900.

demonstration of free cholesterol in the mitochondria, smooth ER and on the
surface of lipid droplets.

As markers of the (smooth) E R, glucose-6-phosphatase and inosine-5'-diphos-
phatase show a specific cytochemical reaction, nevertheless, the second one
presents a more stable binding on the membrane and is considered as the best
marker of microsomes, isolated after differential centrifugation.

When the intracellular volume occupied by the liposomes, mitochondria and
the ER has been determined in the zona fasciculata of guinea-pig, rat and beef
andrenal cortex by stereological analysis and when these results were compared
with the quantities of free and esterified cholesterol, neutral fats and phos-
pholipids, present in the isolated adrenal cortex of the same species, the

following results have been obtained:

In the fasciculata cells of adrenals where the endogenous synthesis of cholesterol remains small (guinea-pig, rat) one finds a great amount of cell space, occupied by lipid droplets containing high quantities of esterified cholesterol and neutral fats.

In contrast, in the adrenal cortex (beef) which presents an important enc genous synthesis of cholesterol the number of lipid droplets is low (less thar 0,6% of the cell volume) corresponding to a very small amount of esterified cholesterol and triglycerides. The quantities of free cholesterol and phospho· lipids are similar in all species studied. The intracellular volume occupied l the smooth ER is high in those cells where the quantity of lipid droplets remains low.

III. Subcellular fractionation

The morphological, stereological and chemical analysis of the subcellulaɪ fractions of the rat adrenal cortex separated by differential centrifugation adapted to this organ allowed us to determine the volumetric participation of each organelle and to measure the exact distribution of cholesterol in each fraction. This method permits a recovery of 85,6% of the total mitochondria ir the mitochondrial fraction, and 91,2% of liposomes in the liposomial fraction. Both fractions demonstrate little contamination with other organelles. The microsomal fraction is also practically pure, but contains only 43,5% of the total tissue "microsomes". The morphological analysis of the fractions allows the demonstration of a distinct liposomal membrane, underlines the close conte between liposomes and certain elements of the endoplasmic reticulum and of mitochondria and confirmes the fact that smooth and granular ER form a single morphological unit.

When the cholesterol distribution among the subcellular fraction of the ɪ adrenal cortex has been studied according to an original technique (7), the following statement could be made:

The redistribution of cholesterol during the centrifugation procedure corresponds partly to the presence of subcellular organelles in other fraction and partly to the absence of a morphologically controlled exchange of molecule Calculation of the redistribution among the three main subcellular fractions revealed that 5,7% of the mitochondrial cholesterol migrated to the microsomes and 6,1% to the liposomes.7,3% of the liposomal cholesterol was discovered in the mitochondria and 0,7% in the microsomes. (About 2/3 of this contamination had no morphological substrate). Microsomes lost 22% of their cholesterol in the mitochondrial fraction and 9,9% in the liposomes, corresponding to a morphologically clear contamination.

IV. Radiochemical data

According to radiochemical analysis of the whole adrenal cortex and of the isolated subcellular organites after a one-shot injection of ^{3}H-cholesterol (CH) the results show, that this molecule enters the cell as free-CH and that there is a continuous transformation to esterified-CH with an initial T1/2 of ± 100 min. The stable esterified-free-CH ratio (90/10) is acheived after 14 hours, and this proportion remains constant at least during 14 days. The incorporation of CH is very rapid into the mitochondria and from the beginning the specific activity of free and esterified-CH is the highest in this subcellular organ. The specific activity of free-CH reaches its peak already after 5 min in the microsomes and remains stable at this level. The lipid droplets show a slowly climbing free-CH activity, presenting the same level as the ER after 24 hours. The greatest part of the labelled esterified-CH is concentrated in the liposomes, nevertheless the specific activity remains 7 times lower than in the mitochondria.

Studies by autoradiography on the ultrastructural level usefully complete these results. During the initial phase the highest labelling level is found in the inner part of the adrenal cortex, especially in the zona reticularis. In all cells of the different zones, the most important radioactivity is identified in the pericapillary section of the cytoplasma.

V. Conclusions

According to all the above mentioned results the following schema of intracellular cholesterol metabolism can be proposed after an one-shot injection of the labelled molecule, which is the standard administration method in the case of isotopic adrenal investigations in man:

The free-CH, injected into the whole organism, enters into the adrenal cortex cells in this form, where it is concentrated in large amounts in the liposomes as esterified-CH, constituting the organic reserves. The ER dispose of a lower and very stable amount of free cholesterol with a slow turn-over, being a structural membrane-cholesterol.

The mitochondria possess the highest level of free and esterified cholesterol activity, which argues in favour of a decisive role of this subcellular organelle in the intracellular metabolism of cholesterol and the other steroids.

The cholesterol enters directly in the mitochondria, being present in both forms of this molecule. The intramitochondrial free-cholesterol seems to be ready directly for the different hydroxylation steps of the normal metabolic pathway. The sterified intramitochondrial-CH might correspond to the dense lipidic granules with 30 to 120 nm diameter (described in the morpholigical chapter) and which could constitute the primairy intracellular reserves, to mobilize in case of stress or hormonal stimulation.

REFERENCES

1. Fawcett DW, Long JA, Jones AL, The Ultrastructure of Endocrine Glands. In: Recent Progress in Hormone Research, Vol. XXV. Astwood EB, (ed), Academic Press, New York, 1969, p. 315.

2. Long JA, Zonation of the Mammalian Adrenal Cortex. In: Handbook of Physiology, Section 7: Endocrinology, Vol. VI: Adrenal Cortex. Blaschko H, Sayers G, Smith AD (eds), American Physiological Society, Washington, 1975, p.13.

3. Malamed S, Ultrastructure of the Mammalian Adrenal Cortex. In: Handbook of Physiology, Section 7: Endocrinology, Vol. VI: Adrenal Cortex. Blaschko H, Sayers G, Smith AD (eds), American Physiological Society, Washington, 1975, p. 25.

4. Idelman S, The Structure of the Mammalian Adrenal Cortex. In: General Comparative and Clinical Endocrinology of the Adrenal Cortex, Vol. II. Chester-Jones J, Henderson IW (eds), Academic Press, New York, London, San Francisco, 1978, p. 1.

5. Nussdorfer GG, Mazzocchi G, Meneghelli V, Cytophysiology of the Adrenal Zone Fasciculata. Int. Rev. Cytol. 55:291, 1978.

6. Frühling J, Correlation entre le métabolisme du cholestérol et la morphologie ultrastructurale dans les cellules de la corticosurrénale du rat. (Thèse). Université Libre de Bruxelles, 1977, p.1.

7. Frühling J, Exchange of Cholesterol between Subcellular Fractions during Differential Centrifugation of Rat Adrenocortical Tissue. In: Separation of Cells and Subcellular Elements. Peeters H (ed), Pergamon Press, Oxford, New York, 1979, p. 91.

THE PHARMACOKINETICS OF SCINTADREN

D.A. TYRRELL

INTRODUCTION

Disorders of the adrenal gland are relatively rare. However, adrenal malfunction can produce a wide variety of symptoms depending upon the pathological
processes involved and accurate diagnosis is essential if irreversible damage
is to be avoided. There are a number of laboratory tests available many of which
are lengthy and expensive investigations. These measurements will frequently
provide a preliminary diagnosis but ultimately a means of visualizing the
adrenals is desirable both for confirmation of the diagnosis and for the
localization of lesions prior to surgery. Thus an effective agent for scintigraphic studies of the adrenals has long been recognized as having great diagnostic value.

Iodocholesterol derivatives for adrenal imaging

The first serious attempts to develop adrenal scanning agents go back to
the late 1960's. A wide variety of compounds were proposed as adrenal imaging
agents but most success has been achieved with radiolabelled steroids which have
been shown to be taken up by the adrenal glands as precursors of steroid
hormones (1). The adrenal glands are rich in cholesterol and in animals (2) and
man (3) it has been demonstrated that (^{14}C) cholesterol is taken from the blood-
stream into the adrenal cortex. In 1969 Counsell et al (4) prepared a derivative
of cholesterol labelled at the C19 carbon atom with ^{131}I. This compound, which
is illustrated in fig. 1 was found to concentrate in the adrenal cortex of dogs
and in 1970 the first scintigrams of human adrenals were obtained with the
material.

In 1974 American (5) and Japanese workers (6) found that an impurity in
(^{131}I)-19-iodocholesterol was concentrated to a greater extent in the adrenal
cortex. Structural analysis of the impurity showed it to be (^{131}I)-6β-iodo-
methyl-19-norcholest-5(10)-en-3β-ol(fig.1). Not surprisingly the name of this

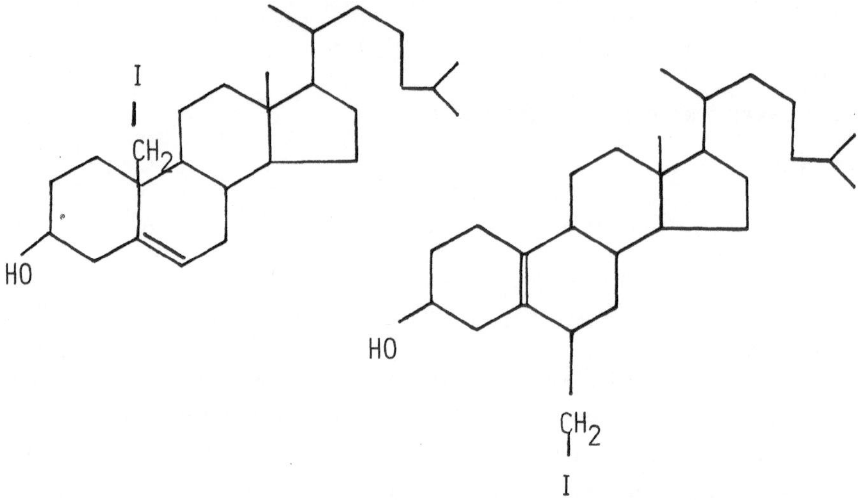

[^{131}I]-19-iodocholesterol

[^{131}I]-6$_\beta$-iodomethyl-19-norcholest-5(10)-en-3$_\beta$-ol

Fig. 1 Iodocholesterol derivatives for adrenal scanning

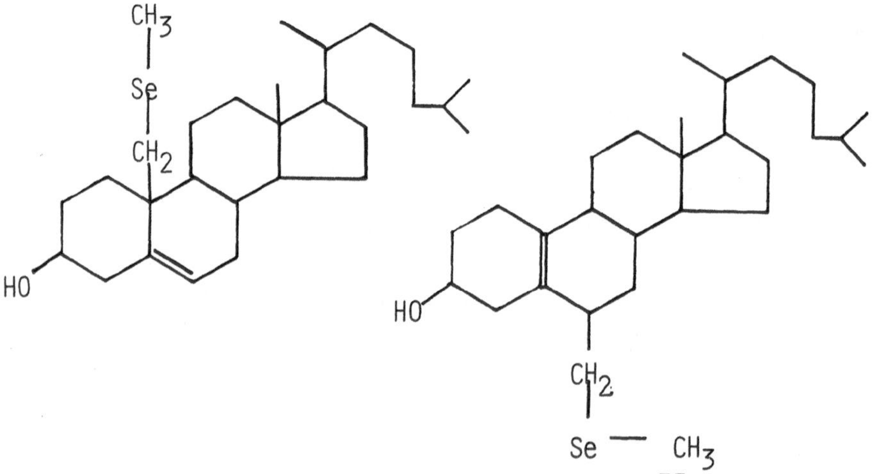

[^{75}Se]-19-methylselenocholesterol

6-β-methyl-[^{75}Se]-selenomethyl 19-norcholest-5(10)-en-3β-ol (Scintadren)

Fig.2 Selenocholesterol derivatives for adrenal scanning

adosterol or (incorrectly) 6-iodocholesterol. Both these iodinated derivatives of cholesterol have subsequently become commercially available.

Selenium labelled steroids for adrenal imaging

At the same time that the iodinated cholesterol derivatives were being developed in the USA and Japan selenium-75 labelled steroids were being investigated at Amersham as potential radiopharmaceuticals. It was realized that selenium-75 had certain advantages over ^{131}I as a label for scintigraphic agents because of the stability of its labelled compounds and its better range of photon energies. Its obvious disadvantage was the 118 day physical half life potentially resulting in greater radiation dose to the patient.

The first ^{57}Se labelled cholesterol derivative produced as a possible adrenal agent was ^{75}Se-19-methyl selenocholesterol followed by 6β-methyl (^{75}Se)-selenomethyl-19-norcholest-5(10)-en-3β-ol (fig.2). A further range of selenocholesterol derivatives was prepared labelled in the 6 and 19 positions. The range comprised butyl, cyclohexyl, benzyl and phenyl seleno derivatives in the 6 position and the 19-methylseleno derivative and its acetate. All these compounds showed high affinity for rat adrenals as shown in table 1. It should be noted that the 5kg dose/g notation is used. This unit means that any value above 0.1 reflects tissue concentration greater than that which would occur if the activity were uniformly distributed throughout the animal.

The 19-methyl selenocholesterol was further assessed in other animal species (7) and showed unexpectedly high uptake in the adrenal medulla in dogs. However, subsequent clinical results with this agent were disappointing. In contrast 6β-methyl selenomethyl-19-norcholest-5(10)-en-3β-ol confirmed its initial promise in animals when tested in humans and was developed commercially as scintadren.

The pharmacokinetics of scintadren in rats

The biodistribution and clearance of scintadren have been extensively investigated in male and female rats. Table 2 shows some typical tissue distribution results following intravenous injection of the agent. There is high uptake by the adrenals 24 hours after injection rising to a peak about 5 days post injection. During the first few days general background remains fairly high but except for the ovaries no other tissue shows appreciable concentration of the agent. This uptake in the overies will be further considered later. The adrenal uptake and background clearance of scintadren compares very well with

TABLE 1

CONCENTRATION OF ^{75}Se CHOLESTEROLS IN RAT ADRENALS

	Y	%kg dose/g (6 days)
'6' compounds RO R=H or acetate CH$_2$SeY	Methyl	14.4
	Methyl(acetate)	12.5
	Butyl	7.5
	Cyclohexyl	3.6
	Benzyl	5.2
	Phenyl	7.3
'19' compounds Y CH$_2$ RO	Methyl	4.6
	Methyl(acetate)	6.3

the iodinated cholesterol derivatives. Fig. 3 shows the whole body clearance scintadren from male and female rats. The main route of excretion is via the liver to the faeces, in which 95% of the injected dose eventually appears. Th exponential components have been fitted to the clearance curves as is demonstrated for female rats in fig. 4. The half lives of the 3 components were approximately equal for male and female rats although the amount of activity cleared as the fast component appears to be greater for males than for female Independant studies by Japanese workers have shown similar tissue distributio and clearance in rats (8).

Tabel 2. Tissue distribution of scintadren in rats

Results are expressed as %kg dose/g M = male F = female									
Tissues		Days after injection							
		1	5	6	10	15	21	25	30
Adrenals	M	4.76	13.98	8.18	9.60	9.04	9.68	9.92	4.00
	F	8.43	16.60	19.68	13.08	10.14	9.41	8.74	7.20
Gonads	M	0.03	0.04	0.02	0.04	0.03	0.02	0.02	0.02
	F	2.67	2.39	3.20	1.87	1.22	0.78	0.99	0.84
Liver	M	0.28	0.07	0.04	0.04	0.02	0.01	0.01	0.01
	F	0.24	0.09	0.07	0.04	0.03	0.02	0.02	0.01
Kidneys	M	0.14	0.10	0.07	0.08	0.05	0.07	0.03	0.02
	F	0.16	0.15	0.15	0.10	0.06	0.04	0.04	0.03
Lungs	M	0.29	0.11	0.08	0.07	0.03	0.03	0.02	0.01
	F	0.38	0.14	0.17	0.07	0.05	0.03	0.03	0.01
Spleen	M	0.31	0.10	0.06	0.06	0.03	0.04	0.01	0.01
	F	0.43	0.13	0.11	0.06	0.04	0.03	0.03	0.02
Blood	M	0.08	0.03	0.02	0.02	0.01	0.01	0.01	0.01
	F	0.10	0.03	0.03	0.02	0.01	0.01	0.01	0.01
Intestine(S)	M	0.18	0.04	0.04	0.02	0.01	0.01	0.01	0.01
	F	0.26	0.04	0.07	0.02	0.03	0.01	0.01	0.01
Intestine(L)	M	–	0.04	–	0.01	0.01	0.01	0.01	–
	F	–	0.06	–	0.02	0.01	0.01	0.01	0.01
Muscle	MF	–	0.03	–	0.12	0.01	–	0.01	–

Clinical studies with scintadren

Scintadren has been effectively used clinically to diagnose a wide range
of adrenal pathologies including Cushings syndrome, Cushings disease, carcinoma,
adrenal insufficiency and phaeochromocytoma. In the case of the latter condition
only indirect evidence for diagnosis is obtained when cortical displacement or
decreased uptake on the side of the tumour is observed. It should be noted that
neither the iodo or seleno cholesterols appear to concentrate in the adrenal
medulla. However, the recent work of Wieland et al (9) with meta iodo benzyl
guanidine offer hope of a significant breakthrough in medullary imaging.

It is not the intention of this paper to discuss the clinical use of
adrenal agents in any detail. However, brief mention should be made of the
distribution and clearance of the agent in volunteers and patients to put into

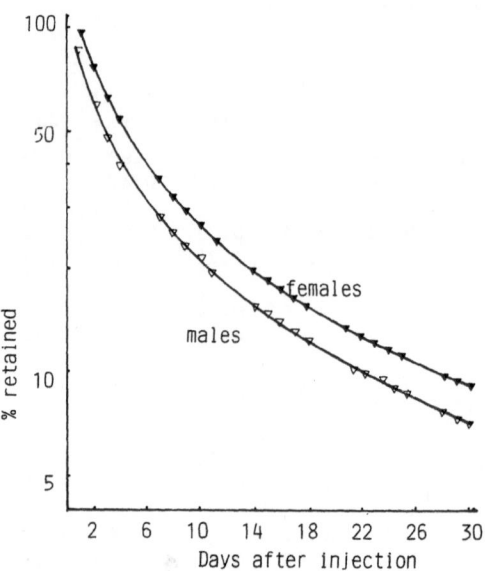

Fig 3 Whole body retention of Scintadren in rats

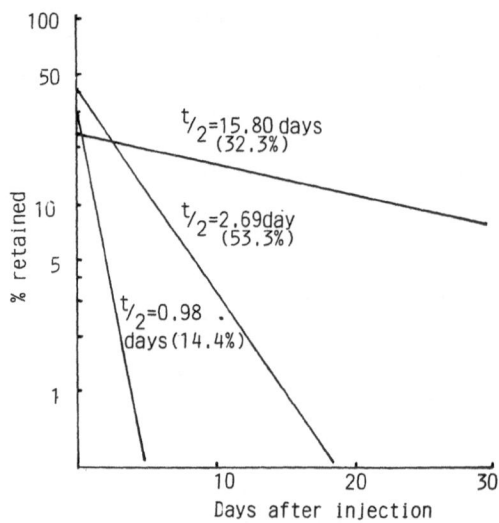

Fig 4 Exponential components of whole body retention
of Scintadren in female rats

Tabel 3. Radiation dosimetry of adrenal scanning agents

	Dose in rads		
	Scintadren 200 µCi	19-^{131}I iodocholesterol 1000 µCi	Adosterol 1000 µCi
Whole body	1.7	1.3	1.2
Liver	2.7	3.4	
Adrenals	4-20	30	150
Ovaries	1.9	1.7	8
Thyroid	-	∿40 blocked	240 unblocked

into context the dosimetry estimates that are discussed in the following section. In humans scintadren is widely distributed throughout the body after injection, the highest concentrations being found in the blood, liver, intestines and adrenal cortex (10). As in rats clearance occurs through the hepatobiliary system leaving the highest concentration in the adrenals after 2-6 days. The estimated half life in the adrenals is variable and lies between 25 and 105 days. About 90% of the injected dose has been cleared from the blood within 6 days and 99% within 35 days. There appears to be a two component clearance from the body with the half lives of the components being approximately 6 and 105 days. Scintigraphic studies of the ovary region have shown that, contrary to the experiments in rats, no activity above background is indicated. These results were confirmed by those obtained in other clinical studies (11,12).

Radiation dosimetry

The clearance data from the rat experiments enabled total absorbed radiation dose to various organs to be calculated and extrapolated to humans. The resulting dose estimates, bearing in mind the high radiation dose obtained from adrenal scanning, were perfectly acceptable with the possible exception of the ovaries. Experience with iodocholesterols had shown a significant drop in gonad uptake when moving from rats to higher animals and this has subsequently proved to be the case for scintadren. Thus dose estimates were revised in the light of the human data and are shown in table 3 in comparison with the iodo-cholesterols. The data shown for adosterol shows a high gonad dose because of the extrapolation of rat data to human estimates. The recommended dose for scintadren in 200 µCi compared to 1 mCi for the iodocholesterols. High adrenal uptake coupled with the superior imaging properties of ^{75}Se compared to ^{131}I account for the lower dose for scintadren. This in turn means that the increas radiation dose resulting from the long half life of ^{75}Se is effectively cancel led out.

A particular advantage of scintadren is its zero dose to the thyroid glan The iodinated materials are both broken down in vivo with the release of free iodine which is taken up by the thyroid.

Conclusions

In current nuclear medicine practice there is a relatively small but well defined need for an agent for scintigraphic visualization of the adrenal corte The major successes for producing such an agent have come in the field of steroids labelled with γ emitting nuclides. Iodo and selenocholesterols have found clinical use in the diagnosis of a range of adrenal pathologies.

Scintadren is a unique ^{75}Se labelled adrenal agent whose pharmacokinetics has been extensively studied in animals and man. In addition to its adrenal localizing properties it offers the following important features:

I. Excellent chemical stability in vitro and in vivo.

II. Long shelf life in the users hands.

III. Improved imaging properties of ^{75}Se over ^{131}I.

IV. No radiation dose to the thyroid.

These additional advantages over the iodocholesterols make scintadren the current agent of choice for adrenal scanning.

REFERENCES

1. Beierwaltes WH et al. Seminars in Nuclear Medicine VIII, p. 5, 1978.

2. Appelgren LE, Acta physiol. scand. suppl. 301, 68:1, 1967.

3. Chobanian AV, Hollander W, J. clin. Invest. 41:1732, 1962.

4. Counsell RE et al. Steroids 16:317, 1970.

5. Sarkar SD et al· J. nucl. Med. 16:1038, 1975.

6. Kojima M, Maeda M, J. chem. Soc. Chemical Communications, p.47, 1975.

7. Sarkar SD, J. nucl. Med. 17:212, 1976.

8. Seto H et al. J. nucl. Med. 16:183, 1979.

9. Wieland DM et al· J. nucl. Med. 22:358, 1981

10. Montz R et al. Nuklearmedizin und Biokybernetik (abstracts). 14 Internatio nale Jahrestagung der Gesellschaft für Nuklearmedizin, September 1976, EV Berlin.

11. Hawkins LA et al. Brit. J. Radiol. 53:883, 1980.

12. Takahashi T et al. Jap. J. nucl. Med. 17:211, 1980.

I-123(131) - METYRAPONE: FACTORS AFFECTING LABELLING

I. ZOLLE, P. ANGELBERGER, W. ROBIEN

INTRODUCTION

H-3-metyrapone has been shown to concentrate in the adrenal cortex (1).
However, data obtained with I-131-metyrapone in rats and dogs indicate that
adrenocortical uptake in the normal adrenal is not sufficient for external
visualization of the gland (2). In patients with Cushing syndrome, adrenal uptake
is increased and the use of I-123 as a radioactive label would permit application
of larger doses of radioactivity. Thus labelling of metyrapone with I-123 in high
specific activity might offer a new radiopharmaceutical for the diagnosis of
hyperfunctioning conditions of the adrenal gland.

I-123 is introduced by halogen exchange in the melt using 4'-bromometyrapone
as a precursor (3). I-123 for Br-exchange without solvent in the melt offers
maximum values for concentration of reactants and temperature and therefore the
highest exchange rate, provided I-123 is available as iodide. It has been reported that I-123 from commercial sources may contain up to 4 additional iodine-
species besides iodide, resulting in lower labelling yields (4). Maximum incor-
oration of radioiodide is however an important aspect because of the high cost
of I-123 and the short physical half-life.

Methods

Labelling: to the I-123-activity, up to 10 mCi in less than 0.1 ml of 0.01N
NaOH, 20 µg of $Na_2S_2O_5$ in 0.005 ml aqueous solution are added. Then 1-2 mg of
4'-bromometyrapone, dissolved in 0.05-0.1 ml ethanol are added and the solvent
evaporated under vacuum at 60°C. The dried reaction mixture is placed into an
oil bath and heated at 165°C for 2 hours. After cooling, the reaction product is
dissolved in 0.5 ml chloroform resp. ethanol for subsequent purification.

Separation of free iodide is performed by:
1. Extraction with an equal volume of an aqueous alkaline solution containing
   0.5 mg KI, 0,5 mg Na-thiosulfate and 1 mg potassiumcarbonate and chloroform.

128

Exchange reaction

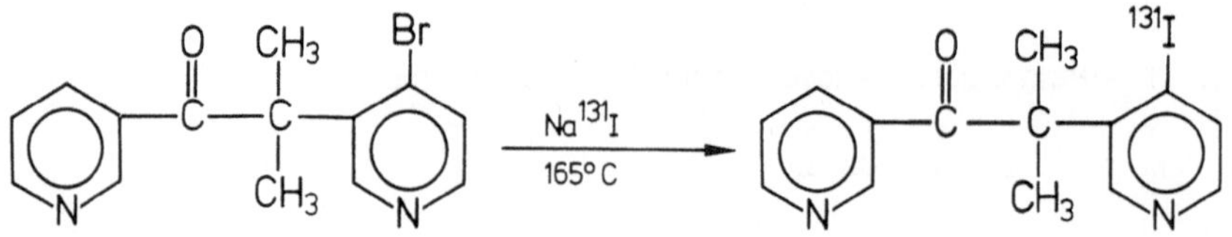

Fig. 1. Chemical structure of 4'-bromometyrapone used for halogen exchange.

Extraction is repeated twice, finally the chloroform phase, containing I-123-metyrapone, is washed once with water.

2. Anion-exchange chromatography on a 9x20 mm Cellex-D column (EtOH-suspension weakly basic DEAE-groups). To assure that unbound iodine is reduced, 0.02 m of a $Na_2S_2O_5$-solution (20 mg/5 ml) is added to the reaction product in 0.5 ethanol. Elution is performed with 2 ml chloroform. After vacuum evaporatic of the solvent, the product is dissolved in ethanol and used as a 5% ethanc solution in saline after membrane filtration.

Radiochemical purity of the product is determined by radio-TLC using Sili Gel F_{254} plates in two solvent systems:

a. Chloroform/methanol (9:1) for identification of the product, $R_f = 0.55$
   - 0.65, single spot by UV-quenching.

b. 1N HCL for determination of free iodide, $R_f = 0.8 = 0.9$,
   R_f for I-123 (131)-metyrapone 0.25-0.35.

Results and discussion

On vacuum evaporation of I-123 solutions, varying amounts of radioactivit (5-39%) were lost, demonstrating variable radiochemical composition and thus t necessity for addition of a reducing agent to convert oxydized forms quantitat: ly into iodide. Of equal significance for successful labelling is the salt content of the I-123 solution. The nucleophilic I for Br-exchange in the melt requires I-123 as no-carrier added iodide with minimum salt content in dry for Concentrations of NaOH corresponding to 0.05 ml of a 0.1N solution have totall prevented labelling. We have used I-123 in aqueous or 0.01N alkaline solution. Any trace of impurity present in the reaction mixture adversely affected the labelling process.

Varying amounts of 4'-bromometyrapone have been used for labelling with I-131. Table 1 shows the percent incorporation obtained when heating for 2 hou

Table 1   INFLUENCE of AMOUNT of Br-METYRAPONE
on LABELING YIELD

Amount (mg)	Labeling (%)
1.5	67.3
1.5	80.8
1.5	54.8
1.8	69.7
2.3	72.5
2.3	83.9
3.5	74.9
4.0	76.5
4.0	72.3
10.0	94.0

There appears to be little correlation between the amount of Br-metyrapone used for labelling and the labelling yield. The major cause for poor halogen exchange has been the formation of I_2 and a too high concentration of NaOH. By keeping the labelling conditions constant we generally obtained 65-75% radiochemical yield.

Besides the chemical requirements it is expected that the heating temperature has the most influence on the exchange rate. Fig. 2 shows the dependance of halogen exchange on temperature and time. At 120°C the duration of heating had little effect on the percent incorporation of label. With increasing temperature labelling increased sharply showing a maximum value at 165°C. 2 hours heating constantly produced higher labelling. 4'-bromometyrapone is resistant to heating showing no degradation products on TLC.

Separation of free iodide from I-123(131)-metyrapone is quantitative both by extraction and ion-exchange chromatography as can be seen in fig. 2. Extraction offers a slight advantage since oxydationproducts are reduced and concentrated in the aqueous phase, while traces of I_2 would not be eliminated by the Cellex-D resin. As a precaution, we have added sodiumpyrosulfite to the reaction product before column chromatography was performed.

Radiochemical purity: Radio-TLC revealed I-123(131)-metyrapone as single spot, identical with the 4'-bromometyrapone standard. No free iodide was measured after separation of the product. After 10-days suspension in saline, 1.0% free iodide was found, indicating a high in vitro stability. When kept in chloroform, only 0.3% unbound radioactivity were present.

Biodistribution: Table 2 shows the relative tissue distribution of I-131-metyrapone obtained 10 and 60 min after intravenous injection in rats. Data are expressed as percent of injected radioactivity per organ, based on a minimum

130

DEPENDENCE OF HALOGEN EXCHANGE ON TEMPERATURE AND TIME

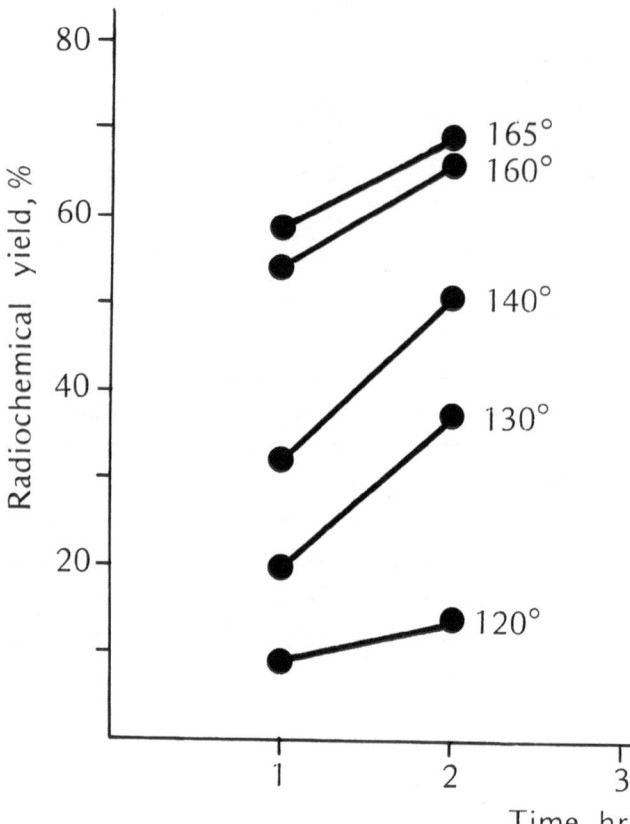

Fig. 2.

of 4 animals. Adrenal uptake of I-131-metyrapone is highest shortly after injection, approximately one half of the radioactivity is eliminated during the
first hour. I-131-metyrapone is concentrated in the liver and excreted via th
intestinal tract. Deiodination is indicated by increased uptake of radioactiv
in stomach, thyroid and kidney. It is apparent that iodide is released slowly
demonstrating a high in vivo stability.

Conclusion

Starting from 4'bromometyrapone, I-123(131)-metyrapone may be obtained i

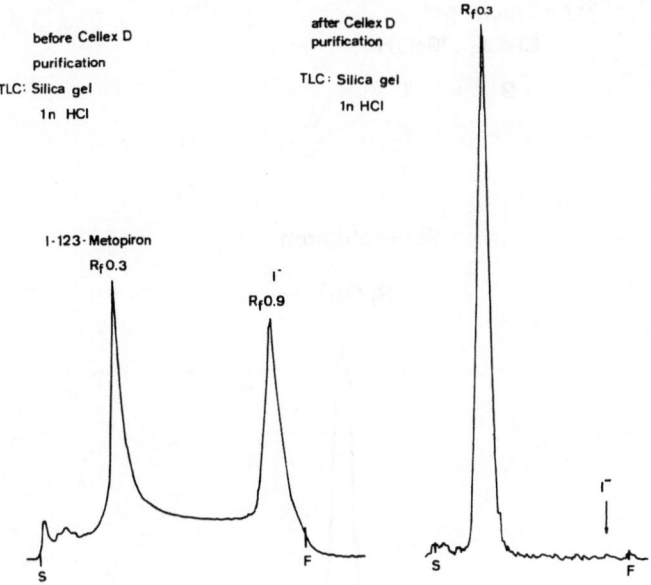

Fig. 3. TLC in 1N HCL. I-123-metyrapone before and after separation of free iodide.

Table 2. Relative tissue distribution of I-131-metyrapone in rats
at 10 and 60 min after injection

(% of injected I-131/organ; mean ± s.e.m.)

Organ	Time 10	60 (min)
Blood	8.17 ± 0.63	5.34 ± 0.66
Heart	0.60 ± 0.09	0.29 ± 0.06
Lung	1.33 ± 0.02	1.22 ± 0.21
Liver	9.85 ± 0.98	7.92 ± 1.16
Intestine	6.77 ± 0.72	23.85 ± 4.41
Pancreas	0.64 ± 0.06	0.32 ± 0.06
Spleen	0.34 ± 0.09	0.22 ± 0.04
Ovary	0.09 ± 0.01	0.06 ± 0.01
Kidney	1.23 ± 0.11	1.57 ± 0.30
Adrenal	0.25 ± 0.03	0.11 ± 0.04
Thyroid	0.06 ± 0.01	0.11 ± 0.04
Stomach	1.91 ± 0.50	2.43 ± 0.30

TLC: Silica gel

CHCl₃ : MeOH

9 : 1

I-123-metopiron

R_f 0.57

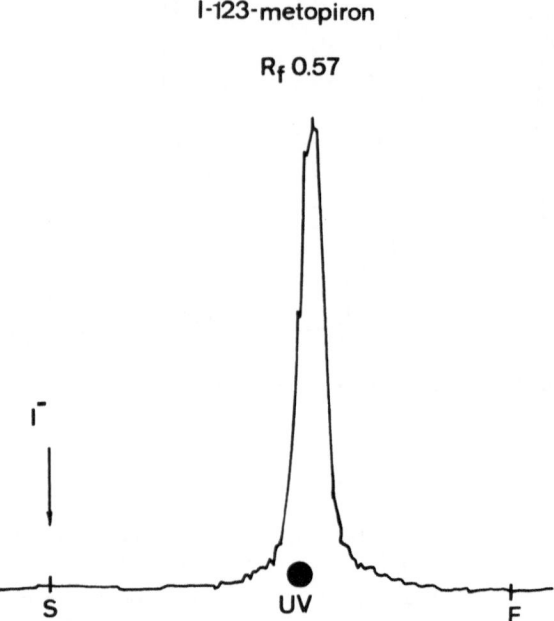

Fig. 3a. TLC in CH1₃/MeOH (9:1) I-123-metyrapone after Cellex-D purification.

in 65-75% radiochemical yield within 3 hours. Using the optimized reaction conditions for labelling and purification of the product, high specific act: ity and high radiochemical purity is obtained. Both in vitro and in vivo st: ity of the radioactive label have been confirmed by radio-TLC and biodistri: tion in rats. It is expected that I-123-metyrapone will find useful clinica: application.

REFERENCES

1. Beierwaltes WH, Wieland DM, Ice RD et al. Localization of radiolabeled inhibitors in the adrenal gland. J. nucl. Med. 17:998, 1976.

2. Zolle I, Robien W, Bergmann H, Höfer R, I-123(131)-metyrapone for imaging of the adrenal cortex. In: Radioaktive Isotope in Klinik und Forschung. Band 15, 2.Teil. Höfer R, Bergmann H (eds), Verlag H. Egermann, Wien, 1982.

3. Robien W, Zolle I, Synthesis of radioiodinated metyrapone. (In preparation).

4. Angelberger P. Wagner-Löffler M, Dudczak R et al. I-123(131)-labelled aliphatic and aromatic fatty acids. Optimized preparation and distribution. In: Radioaktive Isotope in Klinik und Forschung, Band 15, 1.Teil. Höfer R, Bergmann H (eds), Verlag H. Egermann, Wien, 1982.

LOCALIZATION OF RADIOIODINATED ESTROGENIC STILBENES IN
NORMAL AND NEOPLASTIC RAT PROSTATE

L.I. WIEBE, R.J. FLANAGAN, L. GATI, B.C. LENTLE, D.G. McGOWAN

INTRODUCTION

Carcinoma of the prostate is primarily a disease of old age, rarely occur-
ring before the age of 50 but with increasing frequency with advancing age
(1,2). In general this malignancy has a slow growth rate and as a result, the
more aggresive and radical therapy, which would be justifiable in younger
patients and in other diseases, has to be balanced against the potential im-
provement in both quality and quantity of life (3).

In all malignancies, the prognosis is dependent on the stage or degree of
advancement of the malignancy and on the histological grading or degree of
malignancy as judged by microscopic examination. While these two elements are
related in that low stage usually is associated with low histology and high
stage with high grade, there are wide variations and all combinations are
possible (4). In reviewing our data(5), the quantity of tumour clinically detectable, which is not necessarily the same as stage, has an inverse relationship
to the prognosis.

At the two extremes, (a) where there is apparently minimal disease of a low
stage and grade and (b) where there is a great volume of clinically detectable
disease with advanced stage and poor histology, it is desirable to more accurately determine the exact extent of disease. In the former case, no treatment may
be necessary. In the latter case, it is vital that all the known disease be
treated in such a way as to optimise the extent of therapy, that is, treat only
the disease and avoid irradiating normal structures as much as possible.

In younger patients, invasive staging techniques such as laparotomy are
justifiable. In older patients, these techniques constitute a significant hazard
to the patient, possibly greater than the advantages to be gained.

A number of human tumour cells exhibit cytoplasmic or nuclear membrane
receptors for sex hormones, notably the cells of breast and prostatic carcinomata
(6). Not only does this fact afford a potential method for detecting the tumours
in vivo, but it has been found to be important in vitro in the case of planning

breast cancer therapy (7). Thus there are clinical applications which might result from the in vivo detection or characterization of the hormone receptor status of tumours.

However, the non-invasive, scintigraphic diagnosis based on hormone recep labelling present a complex challenge. First, the number of cell receptor site is finite. Thus, a tracer of high specific activity is necessary if there are be signal-to-noise ratios permitting in vivo detection of hormone receptors. Second, the receptors may be avid for androgens or estrogens so that no ubiqui ous tracer may serve in all such contexts. Third, the unbound or non-receptor bound hormone may remain in the blood resulting in further compromise of the signal-to-noise ratios. Fourth, the tracer must retain its biological specific ity. Fifth, the radiolabel must be readily detectable by existing imaging systems, either with or without blood-background substraction. Finally, the radiolabelled hormone must be stable (8).

Against these considerations must be weighed the advantages of a site-specific label (unlike existing non-specific methods of radionuclide tumour imaging such as that using ^{67}Ga-citrate) and one which might not only assist i staging a tumour but also influence the management of the disease and its recurrences as does in vitro hormone receptor assay at present. For these reasons, a hormone receptor label has the potantial for limited but precise an valuable clinical application.

It is therefore desirable to devise a non-invasive technique which would more accurately determine both the local tumour load and also metastatic tumou so that the most effective treatment plan could be devised for each individual patient. To this end, a research program based on the use of estrogenic radio-pharmaceuticals for estrogen-receptor-specific evaluation of metastatic prostat carcinoma has been undertaken.

The selection of an appropriate animal model of prostatic carcinoma for this research was based on a bibliographic survey of the disease in laboratory animals, (9) and on limited local availability of one of the better models, namely the Dunning 3327 adenocarcinoma model in the Copenhagen X Fisher rat. Preliminary data on the uptake of two radioiodinated non-steroidal estrogens by normal prostate, and by this experimental prostatic carcinoma are presented.

MATERIALS AND METHODS

Radioestrogens. Radioiodinated 3-iododiethylstilbestrol diphosphonate (DES-2P-131-I) was prepared by iodination of diethylstilbestrol diphosphonate

(Honvol TM, Frank W. Horner Limited, Montreal), followed by exchange radio-iodination with $Na^{131}I$, as described by Tubis et al (10). The product, which consisted mainly (>90%) of DES-2P-I, but with some DES-1P-I and 3-iododiethyl-stilbestrol (DES-I), (10) had a specific activity of 240 μCi (8.88 MBq) mg^{-1}, or 134 mCi (4.96 GBq)$mmol^{-1}$. This method of preparation has been shown to yield a mixture which contains on the average, 0.4 moles of iodine per mole of estrogen (11). An aqueous solution of the sodium salt (pH8), with a radioactive concentration of 8.-57 mCi ml^{-1}, was used for animal studies.

Radioiodinated 1,2-bis(4-methoxyphenyl)-1-(^{125}I)-iodo-1-propene (Alberta 81.1-125-I) was prepared by exchange labelling of the non-radioactive stilbene with $Na^{125}I$ as described previously (12). The product specific activity was 600 μCi(22.2 MBq)mg^{-1}, or 228 mCi(8.4 GBq)$mmole^{-1}$. This highly lipophilic substance was reconstituted in aqueous ethanol (20%) and Tween 80 (10%), with a final radioactive concentration of 3.75 mCi ml^{-1}. Alberta 81.1 and its mono-methoxy-monohydroxy-(Alta 81.2) and dihydroxy-(Alta. 81.3) analogues labelled with ^{131}I were similarly prepared, according to the literature methods (12), with specific activities of approximately 3.6 Ci(133 GBq)$mmol^{-1}$.

Animal studies were undertaken using normal male Wistar rats (450-600 g), and Copenhagen X Fisher rats (200-250 g) which carried transplanted Dunning 3327H prostatic tumours. The tumour-bearing animals were a gift from Dr J.D. Chapman, Cross Cancer Institute, Edmonton. Because of the limited local availability and the slow growth characteristics of the 3327H tumours, only 3 animals were used; one was pre-treated with estrogen (Honvol TM, 0.66 mg i.v. every second day for a total of 3.3 mg) for 9 days, then left untreated for 5 days prior to dosing with Alberta 81.1-125-I; this animal received an i.v. dose of DES-2P-131-I after an additional 24 hours. The two untreated tumourbearing rats received a single i.v. dose of either DES-2P-131-I or Alberta 81.1-125-I. The estrogen doses were 0.1 ml (857 μCi; 6.4 μmole) for DES-2P-131-I and 0.2 ml (750 μCi; 3.3 μmole) for Alberta 81.1-125-I. Alberta 81.1-131-I, Alberta 81.2-131-I and Alberta 81.3-131-I doses were 1.2 mCi (0.9 nmol) per animal.

Rats receiving the Alberta 81.1/2/3-131-I series were housed in metabolic cages for up to 5 days. Whole-body counts were taken daily for clearance measurements. Animals from each group (81.1; 81.2; 81.3) were sacrificed after 72, 120 and 96 hours respectively for dissection and radioassay of selected tissues. A small number of scintigraphic images were recorded. Rats dosed with Alberta 81.1-125-I and/or DES-2P-131-I were immobilized by light ether anesthesia and monitored for tumour, blood and thyroid radioactivity for 60 min after injection.

Table 1. Whole-body retention of radioactivity in normal rats which received intravenous injections of high specific activity Alberta 81.1-131-I, Alberta 81.2-131-I or Alberta 81.3-131-I.
Data listed represent the mean ± S.D.,   n=6

| Radioestrogen | Percentage of dose retained after i.v. injection (hr) | | | | | |
	0	24	48	72	96	120
81.1	100	53.8± 8.8	32.2±5.7	26.8±4.6	N.D.	N.D.
81.2	100	50.9± 8.9	30.4±3.4	27.5±4.3	24.9±4.4	23.8±4.4
81.3	100	86.2±10.8	64.7±7.3	16.8±1.2	15.9±1.7	N.D.

N.D. - not determined

FIG. 1. TISSUE DISTRIBUTION IN % OF BLOOD VALUE IN NORMAL MALE RATS AFTER 96 HOURS.

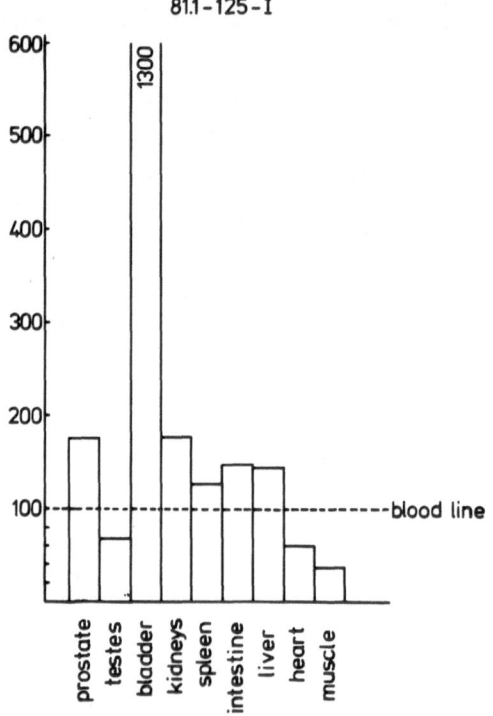

81.1-125-I

Table 2. Tissue distribution of radioactivity in rats after intravenous injection of high specific activity Alberta 81.1-131-I, Alberta 81.2-131-I, or Alberta 81.3-131-I. Data are mean values (dpmx10^{-3}) ± percent S.D. per g of tissue per mCi of injected dose

Tissue	81.1 (72 hr)	dpmx 10^{-3} g tissue^{-1} mCi^{-1} 81.2 (120 hr)	81.3 (96 hr)
blood	0.9 ± 38%	0.3 ± 15%	3.6 ± 23%
adipose	15.2 ± 48%	0.5 ± 33%	2.6 ± 15%
pancreas	7.7 ± 58%	3.3 ± 73%	7.3 ±120%
skin[1]	4.5 ± 23%	0.7 ± 52%	6.1 ± 56%
duodenum[2]	3.6 ±109%	1.4 ± 80%	3.6 ± 16%
stomach[2]	4.1 ± 35%	0.8 ± 40%	2.7 ± 34%
lung	1.7 ± 89%	0.6 ± 45%	3.0 ± 25%
liver	1.7 ± 63%	0.6 ± 37%	5.7 ± 18%
spleen	1.7 ± 34%	0.9 ± 37%	3.2 ± 36%
kidney	1.4 ± 30%	0.6 ± 13%	3.6 ± 18%
prostate	1.1 ± 34%	1.7 ± 69%	2.8 ± 26%
heart	0.8 ± 25%	0.6 ± 51%	3.0 ± 38%
muscle	0.6 ± 45%	0.7 ±110%	7.2 ±164%
testes	0.5 ± 52%	0.3 ± 44%	1.2 ± 18%
brain	0.3 ± 20%	0.5 ± 56%	1.2 ± 13%
thyroid[3]	2700 ± 38%	630 ± 83%	6900 ± 33%

[1] surface contamination not excluded
[2] contents included
[3] not blocked

140

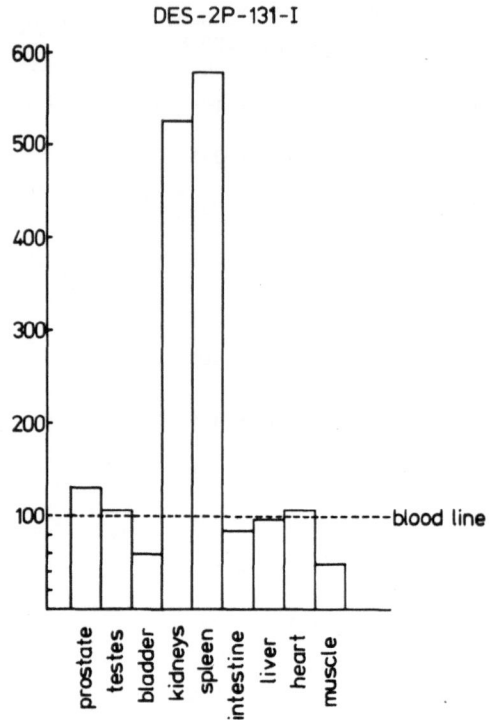

FIG. 2. TISSUE DISTRIBUTION IN % OF BLOOD VALUE
IN NORMAL MALE RATS AFTER 96 HOURS.

DES-2P-131-I

These animals were sacrificed and dissected for tissue radioassay, 96 hours after injection. DES-2P-131-I scintillation images were recorded 10 min, 24 hours and 96 hours after injection.

All radioactive materials were injected via the tail vein or via the su gically-exposed femoral vein. Scintillation images were recorded using a Sea Pho-Gamma IV camera with a pin-hole collimator. A multi-probe monitoring sys with three 2.5 cm collimated NaI detectors and an LSI-11 based data analyser (13) was used to evaluate short-term radioactivity profiles for blood, tumou and thyroid.

FIG. 3. TISSUE DISTRIBUTION IN % OF BLOOD VALUE IN
HONVOL TREATED AND CONTROL TUMOR BEARING
MALE RATS AFTER 96 HOURS.

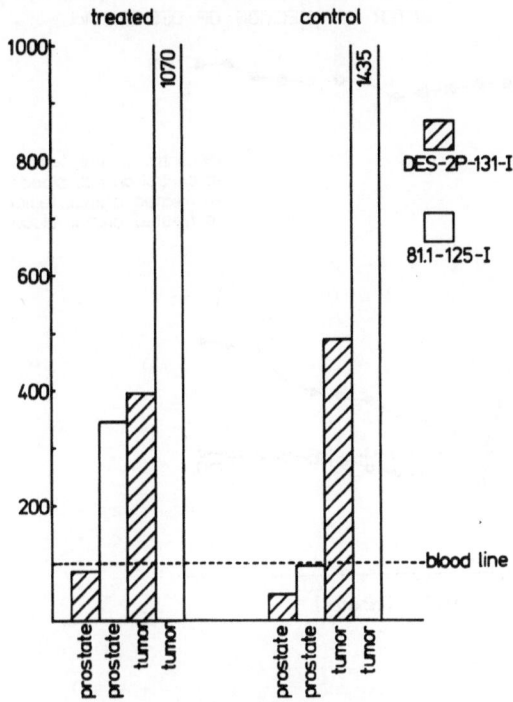

Results

The three-day whole-body retention of Alberta 81.1-131-I represented about
27 percent of the i.v. dose. Similar data were recorded for the dihydroxy and
monohydroxy-monomethoxy analogues of this synthetic estrogen (table I). Radioassay of tissues taken from these animals indicated that a considerable degree
of deiodination had occured, resulting particularly in high thyroid radioactivity. Other tissues which had relatively high radioactivity concentrations
(tissue:blood ratios) included fat (16), pancreas (8.1), stomach (4.3) and
duodenum (3.8) for Alberta 81.1, pancreas (11.4), prostate (6.0), duodenum
(4.8), and spleen (3.3) for Alberta 81,2 and pancreas (2.0), muscle (2.0),

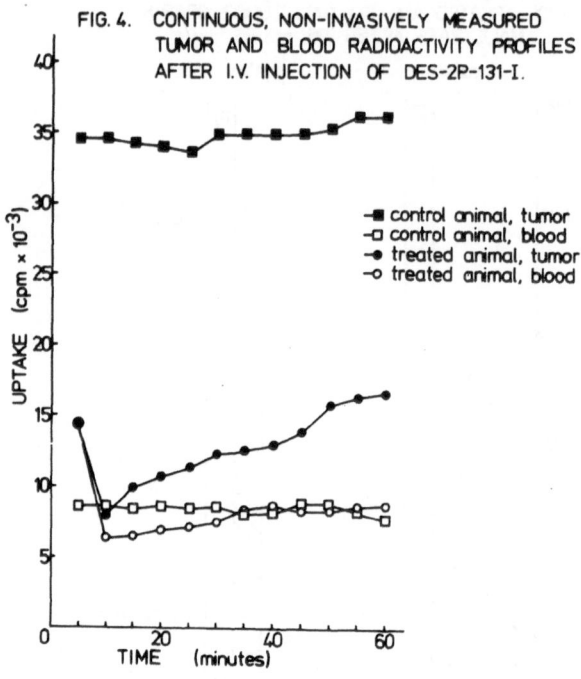

FIG. 4. CONTINUOUS, NON-INVASIVELY MEASURED TUMOR AND BLOOD RADIOACTIVITY PROFILES AFTER I.V. INJECTION OF DES-2P-131-I.

-■ control animal, tumor
-□ control animal, blood
-● treated animal, tumor
-○ treated animal, blood

skin (1.7), and liver (1.6) for Alberta 81.3. Tissue distribution data, norm ized for small dose variations, are presented in table 2. Low specific activ Alberta 81.1-125-I tissue distribution data are expressed in fig. 1; these d are the mean radioactivity concentration values from two animals, expressed a percentage of the blood-concentration; all tissues except the testes, hear and muscle had radioactivity levels above the blood-level, as found with the high specific activity 81.1. Fig. 2 depicts the tissue distribution data for DES-2P-131-I. These data, the mean values from three animals, show high rena and splenic concentrations, and small relative accumulations of radioactivit in the prostate.

Preliminary prostatic tumour and normal prostate uptake data for 81.1-1 and DES-2P-131-I in prostatic-tumour-bearing rats are presented in fig. 3. T

Dunning prostatic tumour showed high uptake of both radioestrogens in non-treated rats and in rats previously treated with therapeutic doses of estrogen. In non-treated tumour-bearing rats there was no indication of concentration of radioestrogen by the prostate. Pretreatment with estrogen induced uptake of 81.1, but not DES-2P, by the prostate. Unfortunately, the small sample (number of animals) in this preliminary study requires further confirmation of these findings.

A limited number of non-invasive measurements were also made. Scintillation imaging with the I-131-labelled estrogens failed to adequately delineate any organ of interest with respect to estrogen receptor labelling. Similarly, the use of strategically-positioned scintillation detectors failed to show any significant changes in the count rate over any tissue from 5 to 50 min after injection of Alberta 81.1-125-I. These studies did show that the relative tumour : blood-ratio observed upon dissection after 96 hours was already evident after 5 min. In the case of DES-2P-131-I similar results were found for the untreated rat. In the treated rat, however, the tumour : blood-ratios were near unity for 10 min, after which the tumour radioactivity increased steadily over the 60 min counting period (fig. 4).

Discussion

The search for a radiolabelled marker of estrogen receptors, which would effectively delineate the receptor-containing tissues by non-invasive observation, has been characterized by almost universal frustration and limited achievement. Early studies with tritium-labelled natural estrogens (14) led to the introduction of gamma-emitting estrogens for non-invasive diagnosis. Included among the first compounds to be synthetized and tested were DES-2P-131-I (10); now the list includes fluorine-18 labelled estrone and estradiol (15), radiobrominated (16) andradioiodinated (17) estradiols and others (18,19). The basis of diagnosis using this approach is the basis of action of the estrogen. As is evident upon consideration of scheme 1, only a small portion of any (administered) estrogen will be able to find a specific estrogen receptor, the largest part of the dose being lost to excretion, metabolism, and intracellular and extracellular binding which may be specific or non-specific but which nonetheless is not true receptor binding. Furthermore, should the diagnostic estrogen "see" one is the finite number of true receptors, that receptor may be occupied by an endogenous estrogen which prevents or slows uptake. Thus, the need for a very high specific activity radiodiagnostic is apparent, a specific activity estimated

A Model For Estrogen Action

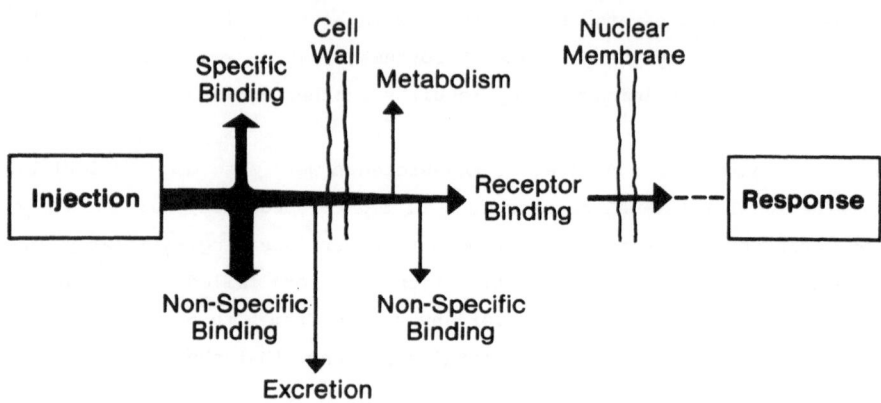

to be 1000 Ci/mmole (8) or higher. Furthermore, a strong affinity for the rece
tor is mandatory so that once in place, the estrogen will remain firmly bound
until most or all of the non-receptor bound material has been cleared from the
body. Meanwhile, it must remain intact in the face of chemical and enzymatic
assault.

The designs of suitably-labelled gamma-emitting estrogens are based on th
needs of a receptor model which has high affinity and specificity for natural
estrogens such as esterone and estradiol. Many estrogenic substances fit the
physical criteria of this model well, and are potent estrogens; diethylstilbestrol (DES) for example, has estrogenic activity of the same order as estrad
(20). The introduction of bulky lipophilic halogen atoms such as bromine or
iodine frequently reduce the biopotency of these estrogens, as in the case of
DES, where iodination in the 3-position to make DES-2P-131-I, reduces the estr
genic potency by almost two orders of magnitude (21). Furthermore, introductio
of iodine in the 3-position of DES may prevent binding with estradiol binding
protein (22). Alberta 81.1 would, on the basis of known structure-activity
relationships (SAR) (21), be expected to have a biopotency approaching that of
DES itself. Although phosphatase activity in the prostate is higher than in mo
tissues, (23) thereby making a phosphate ester of the estrogen a carrier for
local deposition of the estrogen in the prostate, its main advantages may lie
the ease of formulation as an aqueous intra venous dose form, and rapid urina

elimination of unbound drug. The methoxy substituents on DES, conversely, contribute to the already significant lipophilicity of these compounds.

Before addressing the experimental observations presented above, it is also necessary to consider the current status of normal and neoplastic prostatic tissue as specific targets for estrogens, and to examine the animal tumour models available for pre-clinical studies. The existence of an estrogen receptor in human prostatic tissue remains the subject of debate, with positive (24,25) and negatieve (26) reports in the literature. Although the mechanism may remain obscure, the effectiveness of estrogens in controlling prostatic carcinomas is well established (27).

The Noble (Nb) rat prostatic adenocarcinoma (28) and the Dunning 3327 prostatic adenocarcinoma (29) were the two animal prostatic tumour models available in limited supply on our campus. Both of these tumour lines appear to be appropriate models for the study of the human condition, demonstrating some histological and biochemical similarities including responsiveness to hormones, and undergoing metastasis; a number of sublines of each are known (30-32). The selection of the Dunning tumour model for present studies was based in part on reports of the presence and/or estrogen-inducibility of both estrogen and progesterone receptors (33,34).

In the present investigation, a new iodine-containing synthetic estrogen (12) labelled with radioiodine was prepared and tested as the dimethoxy, mono-methoxy-monohydroxy, and dihydroxy forms. Although all three forms had been shown to be stable in vitro, whole-body clearance data (table 1), scintillation imaging and dissection studies (table 2) all indicated extensive deiodination in vivo. This was most evident in stomach and thyroid radioactivity levels. In other respects, the in vivo distribution of i.v. doses of these compounds, at high specific activities, were similar to those reported for DES-2P-131-I (35). The relatively high uptake of the Alberta 81.-131-I series of compounds by pancreas (pancreas : blood = 8), 11 and 2 for 81.1, 81.2 and 81.3 respectively) was of particular interest in the light of the known presence of estrogen receptors in that organ (37). The doubly protected (dimethoxy; Alberta 81.1) stilbene reflected its enhanced lipophilicity through high concentrations in adipose tissue. At lower specific activities (figs. 1 and 2), there were only small differences among the relative distributions of DES-2P-131-I and Alberta 81.1-125-I, except for the renal and splenic uptakes which were much higher for the former.

In the small number of Dunning 3327H tumour-bearing rats studied, there was no evidence of an early (e.g. within 60 min) enhanced uptake of either DES-2P-

131-I or Alberta 81.1-125-I above the initial (perfusion) level. However, the:
was an apparent gradual uptake of DES-2P-131-I derived radioactivity by the
prostatic tumour during the first hour after injection (fig. 4) into the
estrogen pre-treated rat.

The effect of estrogen pre-treatment had no apparent influence on the
uptake of either radioestrogen by the transplanted prostatic tumour, but did
enhance the uptake of Alberta 81.1-125-I by the "normal" prostate of an anima:
bearing a transplanted prostatic tumour (fig. 3). In both instances, the tran:
planted tumours were found to have much higher concentrations of radioactivit
than either blood (>10 for 81.1-125-I; >4 for DES-2P-131-I) or normal prostat
In the estrogen-pre-treated animal, Alberta 81.1-125-I concentrations in the
prostate approached those for DES-2P-131-I in the prostatic tumour. These preliminary findings, if reflective of true estrogen receptor binding, are in
keeping with previously reported unsuccessful attempts to induce estrogen
receptors in the Dunning 3327 tumour (34), but are in keeping with the reporte
normal presence of estrogen receptors in the tumour.

The preliminary data reported here require additional substantiation and
clarification. However, these data together with other literature do not suppc
any optimism over the eventual applicability of a radioestrogen-based non-
invasive diagnostic procedure for benign prostatic hyperplasia nor prostatic
neoplasia. This is particularly the case if the radiopharmaceutical or any
radioactive part thereof is cleared from the body either fecally or via the
urinary tract, with an appreciable (relative to the half-life of the radionuclide) half-life. However, the prospects for detection and/or evaluation of
metastastic prostatic tissues located elsewhere in the body remain much more
promising.

Acknowledgements

The authors wish to thank Drs. Nick Bruchovsky, Paul Rennie and Bill
McBlain for their interest and helpful discussion, Dr. J.D. Chapman for the
donation of Dunning 3327H tumour-bearing rats, and Dr. Wendy Gati and Ms.
Lindsay McQueen and Mr. Igor Shaskin for technical assistance. This research
was supported by grant H-1 of the Alberta Heritage Trust Fund : Applied
Research-Cancer.

REFERENCES

1. Mostofic F, Leestma J, Lower urinary tract and male genitalia. In: Pathology, Vol. I, 6th ed. Anderson W (ed), Mosby, St. Louis, p. 850, 1971.

2. Whitemore WF, jr, The natural history of prostatic cancer. Cancer 32:1104, 1973.

3. Corriere JN, jr, Cornog JL, Murphy JJ, Prognosis in patients with carcinoma of the prostate. Cancer 25:911, 1970.

4. Gleason DF, Histologic grading and clinical staging or prostatic cancer. In: Urologic Pathology: The prostate. Tannenbaum M (ed), Lea & Febiger, Philadelphia, p. 171, 1977.

5. McGowan DG, unpublished.

6. Bruchovsky N, Rennie P, Van Doorn E, Steroid receptors in cancer. Mod. Med. of Canada 31:914, 1976.

7. DeSombre ER, Smith S, Block GE et al. Prediction of breast cancer response to endocrine therapy. Cancer Chemother. Rep. 58:513, 1974.

8. Krohn KA, The search for a gamma-emitting estrogenic ligand. J. nucl. Med. 21:593, 1980.

9. Rivenson A, Silverman J, The prostatic carcinoma in laboratory animals. Invest. Urol. 16:468, 1979.

10. Tubis M, Endow JS, Blahd WH, The preparation of ^{131}I labeled diethylstilbestrol diphosphate and its potential use in nuclear medicine. J. nucl. Med. 6:184, 1967.

11. Mende T, Wollny G, Gens J, On the use of radioiodine-labeled diethylstilbestrol diphosphate as a scanning agent of the liver. Nucl. med. Comm. 3,1982 in press. See: Wollny G, Gens J, Mende T, Jahresbericht des Bereiches Kernchemis des ZFK Rossendorf, 340-60, 1977.

12. Flanagan RJ, Lently BC, McGowan DG, Wiebe LI, α-Halostilbenes related to diethylstilbestrol. J. rad. Chem. 65, 81, 1981.

13. Ediss C, McQuarrie SA, In-house design and construction.

14. Ullberg S, Bengtsson G, Autoradiographic distribution studies with natural estrogens, Acta endocr. 43:75, 1963.

15. Eakins MN, Palmer AJ, Waters SL, Studies in the rat with ^{18}F-4-fluoroestradiol and ^{18}F-4-fluoro-oestrone as potential prostate scanning agents: comparison with ^{125}I-2-iodo-oestradiol and ^{125}I-2,4-diiodo-oestradiol. Int. J. appl. Radiat. Isotopes 30:395, 1979.

16. McElvany KD, Katzenellebogen JA, Senderoff SG, Siegel BA, Welch MJ, Tissue distribution, clearance rates and radiation dosimetry of 16α(Br-77)-bromo-estradiol-17β. J. nucl. Med. 22:19, 1981.

17. Gatley SJ, Shaughnessy WJ, Inhorn L, Lieberman LM, Studies with 17β(16α(^{125}I) Iodo)-Estradiol, an estrogen receptor-binding radiopharmaceutical, in rats bearing mammary tumors. J. nucl. Med. 22:459, 1981.

18. Mazaitis JK, Gibson RE, Komai T, Eckelman WC, Francis B, Reba RC, Radioiodinated estrogen derivatives, J. nucl. Med. 21:142, 1980.

19. Heiman DF, Senderoff SG, Katzenellebogen JA, Neeley RJ, Estrogen receptor based imaging agents. 1. Synthesis and receptor binding affinity of some

aromatic and D-ring halogenated estrogens. J. med. Chem. 23:994, 1980.

20. Dodds EC, Lawson W, Noble RL, Biological effects of the synthetic oestrogenic substance 4:4'-dihydroxy-α:diethylstilbene. Lancet 1:1389, 1938.

21. Grundy J, Artificial estrogens. Chem. Rev. 57:281, 1957.

22. Komai T, Eckelman WC, Johnsonbaugh RE, Mazaitis A, Kubota H, Reba RC, Estrogen derivatives for the external localization of estrogen-dependent malignancy. J. nucl. Med. 18:360, 1977.

23. Marberger H, Riedesel RD, Anderson DO, Malek LH, A comparative study of phosphatase activities of various human tissues. J. Urol. 75:857, 1956.

24. Hawkins EF, Nijs M, Brassine C, Tagnon HJ, Steroid receptors in the human prostate. 1. Estradiol-17β binding in human prostatic hypertrophy. Steroi 26:458, 1975.

25. Bashirelahi N, O'Toole JH, Young JD, A specific 17β-estradiol receptor in human benign hypertrophic prostate. Biochem. Med. 15:254, 1976.

26. Eckman P, Snochowski M, Dahlberg E, Bression D, Hogberg B, Gustafsson JA, Steroid receptor content in cytosol from normal and hyperplastic human prostates. J. clin. Endocr. Metab. 49:205, 1979.

27. Fergusson JD, Castration and oestrogen therapy. In: Endocrine Therapy of malignant disease. Stoll BA (ed), Saunders, London, p. 247, 1972.

28. Noble RL, Hochachka B, King D, Spontaneous and estrogen produced tumors i Nb rats and their behavior after transplantation. Cancer Res. 35:766, 197

29. Dunning WF, Prostatic cancer in the rat. Nat. Cancer Inst. Monograph, 12: 351, 1963.

30. Drago JR, Ikeda RM, Maurer RE, Goldman LB, Tesluk H, The Nb rat: prostati adenocarcinoma model. Invest. Urol. 16:353, 1979.

31. Seman G, Meyers B, Bowen JM, Dmochowski L, Histology and ultrastructure o the R-3327 C-F transplantable prostate tumor of Copenhagen-Fisher rats. Invest. Urol. 16:231, 1978.

32. Collins JM, Bagwell CB, Block NL, Claflin AJ, Orvin GL, Pollack A, Stover Flow cytometric monitoring of R3327 rat prostate carcinoma. Invest. Urol. 19:8, 1981.

33. Heston WDW, Menon M, Tananis C, Walsh PC, Androgen, estrogen and progesterone receptors of the R3327 Copenhagen rat prostatic tumor. Cancer Lett 6:45, 1979.

34. Ip MM, Milholland RJ, Rosen F, Functionality of estrogen receptor and Tamoxifen treatment of R3327 Dunning rat prostatic adenocarcinoma. Cancer Res. 40:2188, 1980.

35. Mende T, Wollny G, Gens J, Schubert J, Verteilung und kinetik von Diaethy stilbostroldiphosphat(Cytonol) nach intravenoeser injektion. Europ. J. nuc Med. 4:133, 1979.

36. Mende T, Hennig K, Wollny G, Gens J, Experimentelle untersuchungen über di Verteilung von intravenoes injiziertem jodmarkiertem Cytonol (diaethylstil bostroldiphosphat). Z. Urol. u. Nephrol. 71:529, 1978.

37. Tesone M. Chazenbalk GD, Ballejos G, Charreau EH, Estrogen receptor in rat pancreatic islets. J. Steroid Biochem. 11:1309, 1979.

38. Dahlberg E, Snochowki M, Gustafsson JA, Comparison of the R-3327H rat prostatic adenocarcinoma to human benign prostatic hyperplasia and metastatic carcinoma of the prostate with regard to steroid hormone receptors. The prostate, 1:61, 1980.

BRAIN

PHYSIOLOGY AND PATHOPHYSIOLOGY OF CEREBRAL BLOOD FLOW

G.F. FUEGER AND E. OTT

Peripheral influences

The maintenance of normal cerebral function and perfusion depends on the effectiveness of the cardiovascular system, on the volume and constitution of the blood itself and on the function of the lung, of the liver and of the kidneys. Tissue perfusion is made possible by cardiac contraction, which develops the force needed for the propagation of blood within the blood vessels by resistance to flow provided by changes in the arteriolar diameters of the vascular system, by the amount of blood within the active circulation, by the constitution of the blood, such as the number of red blood cells, the viscosity, the pH, the concentration of vasoactive substances and metabolites. The lung facilitates the exchange of O_2 and CO_2. The liver and kidney provide energy carrying metabolites and eliminate metabolic waste substances.

Cardiac output (1)

Cardiac output is defined as the volume of blood pumped into the general circulation per unit of time. The ratio of blood volume to cardiac output equals the mean circulation time. The ability of the heart to maintain its pumping function is a major requirement as well as the availability of an adequate blood volume. The factor which limits cardiac output (under normal resting conditions) is not the pumping ability of the heart but the amount of venous return, i.e. the ability of the blood to return to the heart (this, of course, is controlled by the peripheral vasculature, which by dilatation or opening of arteriovenous anastomoses enables a certain volume of the cardiac output to flow through its branches).

Under physiological conditions cardiac output is determined by the metabolic needs of peripheral tissues and venous return and normally the cardiac output is maintained at levels greater than the needs of the tissues would actually require. Under pathological conditions which may reduce the pumping ability of the heart (myocardial infarction, cardiac valvular disease, myocard-

itis, myocardiopathy, cardiac insufficiency, congestive failure, cardiac
arrhythmia), the heart becomes the limiting factor for cardiac output and hence
for tissue perfusion in general and for brain perfusion in particular.

Conditions which interfere with the venous return will reduce cardiac output likewise and therefore cause diminution of global blood flow which may be
accompanied by certain clinical symptoms such as faintness or syncope.

The peripheral vascular system

The systemic circulation is arranged in a series of parallel channels
joining the arterial and venous sides. There are major parallel circuits throuc
the individual organs (and regions) and lesser ones within the tissues themselves. The major parallel pathways are: coronary,cerebral, renal, portal and thos
through skin, muscle, skeleton and other tissues; the circulation through the
spleen is in turn a parallel pathway alongside a part of the portal circulation
The lesser parallel circulatory circuits are the arterial-venous capillaries an
arterial-venous anastomoses. The former, when patent, permit blood to by-pass
portions of the capillary bed whereas the latter provide an alternative shorter
path of low resistance between the arterial and venous sides of the systemic
circuit. Thus alterations in the pattern of blood flow may be caused by changes
in the diameter (radius) and length, respectively, of the channels. The left
ventricle forces blood into the arterial reservoir while the arterials limit it
rate of escape.

Peripheral vascular resistance is associated with the contractile state of
the arterioles. Their muscle fibers possess a basal level of tone thought to be
determined by blood-borne materials. They can actively dilate or contract. The
arterioles possess rings like smooth muscle sphincters. The innervation of the
arterioles in the body may have reciprocal innervation to the left ventricle.
Vascular resistance is overwhelmingly determined by the radius of the blood
vessels and the physical proportion of the blood. Caliber-, Diameter-Radius is
altered by passive elastic components, by active smooth muscle elements of the
vessel walls, and by pathologic alterations causing stenosis or obstruction:
Active reversible changes in resistance are brought about by neurogenic influences, or vasomotor reactions to changes in blood pressure or metabolic needs
of the tissue. The fraction of cardiac output received by a tissue is. determine
by the local resistance of the vascular bed of that tissue. Normally cardiac
output ranges around 15 l/min.

Autonomic nervous regulation

The sympathetic nervous system is responsible for rapid circulatory adjustments in response to a variety of stressful physiological and pathological conditions such as temperature changes, hemorrhagic shock, hypoxia and emotional stress. A sympathetic discharge causes an adjustment of the peripheral circulation by the regulation of vascular resistance in each organ which, in turn, governs the fraction of cardiac output supplied to that organ, or, in other words, the perfusion of that organ. There are several components of the sympathetic nervous system. The adrenergic component, which has norepinephrine as a neurotransmitter, is the major pathway, and it moderates the level of vasoconstriction in each vascular bed. Other sympathetic components mediate vasodilatation through the release of either acetylcholine or histamine.

Adrenergic component

The resistance of each vascular bed is determined by the density of the sympathetic adrenergic innervation, by the responsiveness of the resistance vessels to the neurotransmitter norepinephrine, ans by the frequency of efferent sympathetic discharge.

The activation of sympathetic efferent vasoconstrictor pathways is not uniform. Activation of an afferent input, for example through stimulation of chemoreceptors, may result in a selective activation of efferent sympathetic fibers so that vasoconstriction may occur in some areas and vasodilation in others. Such a differential response is likely to modify tissue perfusion in each organ even if cardiac output remains constant.

Inhibition of neurogenic vasoconstriction is observed following stimulation of arterial mechanoreceptors (baroreceptors) during a rise in pressure or stimulation of myocardial receptor during an acute increase in cardiac size. Depending on the degree of inhibition of vasoconstrictor tone in different circulations such reflexes may cause a redistriburion of flow to various organs.

The autonomous nervous system controls the level of cardiac output, blood pressure and tissue perfusion pressure, but also determines the relative distribution of cardiac output upon the various tissues. During sleep or other vagal preponderance there may be a relative decrease in the cerebral fraction of cardiac output without actual cardiac failure as a consequence of autonomic dysfunction. If associated with arterial stenoses this may result in temporary regional ischemia. Vagal stimulation may slow or arrest cardiac contractions, weaken the force of the heartbeat, depress conduction within the heart, or reduce markedly the refractory period of auricular musculature.

The parasympathetic system is organized mainly for discrete and localized discharge and not for mass responses. It slows down the heart rate, lowers the blood pressure, stimulates the gastro-intestinal secretions and movements, aid absorption of nutrients, protects the retina from excessive light, and empties the urinary bladder and rectum. The anabolic purposes of parasympathetic pre-ponderance are associated with a lowered heart rate and a shift of the fractic al relative distribution of cardiac output in favour of the digestive function The gastro-intestinal tract would receive a larger fraction of cardiac output the expense of the fractions supplied to the coronary, cerebral and muscular, dermal blood flow. In order for the brain to be protected against too great re ductions of global blood there is an autonomous cholinergic control of the reactivity of the cerebral vessels to increased CO_2 (2, 3, 4).

Regulation of cerebral blood flow

In considering blood flow to the brain it is necessary to differentiate between perfusion to the whole of the brain, to one hemisphere, or to a region Global cerebral blood flow may be diminished for a variety of reasons, such as diminished venous return to the heart, impairment of the pumping function of t heart, inadequate quality of the blood (polycythemia), hypertensive encephalo-pathy or severely increased intracranial pressure (see tables 1 and 2).

Table 1: Causes of diminished global brain perfusion

Diminished venous return
    Hypovolemia
    Inadequate vasoconstrictor mechanism
        Vasovagal (vasodepressor) syncope
        Postural hypotension
        Primary autonomic insufficiency (SHY-DRAGER)
        Neurologic al diseases.
        Cardial sinus syncope

Mechanical impairment (of venous return)

> Valsalva's meneuver, cough, arterial mysome

> Ball valve thrombus

Impairment of pumping fuction

> Bradyarrhythmia's

>> A-V-block with Stokes-Adams-attack,

>> ventricular asystole,

>> Sinusbradycardia, sino atrial block, sinus arrest

> Tachyarrhythmia's

> Obstruction to flow

>> Aortic stenosis, hypertrophic subaortic stenosis,

>> pulmonia, stenosis, primary pulmonary

>> hypertension, pulmonary embolism

> Cardiac tamponade

> Myocardial infarction

Inadequate quality of the blood

> Anemia, acidosis, hypokapnia due to hyperventilation,

> hypoglycemia, polycythemia

Cerebro-vascular diseases

> Hypertensive encephalopathy

> Cerebral infarct

> Subarachnoid hemorrhage

Increased intracranial pressure

Intrinsic regulation of cerebral blood flow (CBF)

Adequate function of the CBF regulatory mechanism is needed as a prerequisite for satisfactory cerebral blood flow. The influence of systemic conditions upon global cerebral blood flow needs to be compensated. This is mediated by the autonomic nervous system (fractional cardiac output to brain) and by the intrinsic regulation of CBF. Local needs of the tissue metabolism are reacted to by the cerebral blood vessels upon local chemical or metabolic stimuli. The effectiveness of such local stimuli is mediated by the autonomous nervous system which enhances or restricts the ability of the cerebral blood vessels to dilate or constrict, and by autoregulation.

Conceptually the regulation of blood flow can be accomplished, in physical

Table 2: Change in Regional Blood Volume

Regional Blood Volume		Circulation Time		Blood Flow	
120	(BLV)	6	(BLV)	20	Base Line Conditions
132	(+ 10%)	6	(BLV)	22	Vasodilation
108	(- 10%)	6	(BLV)	18	Vasoconstriction
120	(± 0%)	5	(- 15%)	24	Increased Pulse Rate
120	(± 0%)	7	(+ 15%)	17	Lowered Pulse Rate
132	(+ 10%)	5	(- 15%)	26,4	
132	(+ 10%)	7	(+ 15%)	18,8	
108	(- 10%)	5	(- 15%)	21,6	
108	(- 10%)	7	(+ 15%)	15,4	

Change relative to Base Line Value (BLV)

terms, by a change in regional blood volume or circulation time. Assuming a regional blood volume od 120 ml and a circulation time of 6 sec the blood flov amounts to 20 ml/sec, since

$$\text{Cerebral Blood Flow (ml/sec)} = \frac{\text{Regional Blood Volume (ml)}}{\text{Circulation Time (sec)}}$$

This consideration shows that a change in blood flow can be brought abou either by a change in the regional blood volume or a change in the circulatio time or both. Thus an increase in cerebral blood flow is accomplished by increasing the regional blood volume, i. e. vasodilation, or by shortening of t] circulation time, i. e. increased pulse rate, or both.

A mere physiologically oriented concept demands the dependence of blood flow from perfusion pressure and cerebrovascular resistance

$$\text{Cerebral Blood Flow (ml/min)} = \frac{\text{Cerebral Perfusion Pressure}}{\text{Cerebrovascular Resistance}}$$

$$= \frac{CPP}{CVR}$$

Metabolic control of cerebral blood flow

Inhalation of CO_2 causes an average increase of cerebral blood flow. If the arterial p CO_2 is increased to 70 mm Hg or above, the arterioles become dilated maximally. Autoregulation is abolished and CO_2 narcosis usually supervenes when arterial pCO_2 increases above this level. The response to the inhalation of CO_2 mixture is rapid, occuring within a few seconds. Mean arterial blood pressure increases slightly during inhalation of low CO_2 gas mixtures and accounts for the small percentage of increase in cerebral perfusion pressure. After cessation of CO_2 inhalation CBF continues to increase for one minute due to increased tissue pCO_2 within the brain.

Hyperventilation causes a fall of both alveolar CO_2 and arterial pCO_2, while the arterial pO_2 and arterial saturation with O_2 (SaO_2) increase. The cerebral vessels constrict and CBF decreases to low levels if hyperventilation is continued.

Autoregulation of CBF

Autoregulation of CBF is defined as the inherent property of the brain to maintain constant cerebral blood flow despite changes in perfusion pressure. Autoregulation is the property of cerebral vessels to respond to changes in perfusion pressure in order to maintain a constant cerebral perfusion rate. A drop in mean arterial blood pressure elicits dilatation of the cerebral vessels, increased systemic blood pressure causes vasoconstriction. Global cerebral blood flow is maintained at normal levels by changes in regional blood volume by the mechanism of cerebral vascular autoregulation within a bandwidth of approx 65 and 180 mm Hg. (5)

In post anoxic and post ischemic states such as within the first few days following an acute cerebrovascular accident the autoregulation is lost whereby CBF becomes dependent on cerebral perfusion pressure. Autoregulation is also lost following diffuse or localized brain damage such as respiratory encephalo-pathies, severe metabolic acidosis, and presumably in other conditions characterized by derangement of cellular metabolism and acidosis.

Neurogenic control

A regulatory cholinergic center in the brain stem governs the extent to which the cerebral vessels will respond to local tissue CO_2 and other metabo: stimuli (6, 2). In baboons the injection of Atropine into one of the vertebra arteries inhibited the cholinergic activity of the vasomotor regulatory cent in the brain stem so that inhalation of vasodilating 5% CO_2 elicited a lesse response in CBF than was observed before Atropine injection. The reduction o: global cerebral blood flow by hyperventilation due to vasoconstriction was accentuated by the injection of Atropine into the vertebral arteries. The opposite effects of 5% CO_2 inhalation and hyperventilation were observed afte injection of Neostigmine into one of the vertebral arteries.

Alterations of cerebral blood flow
Anatomical considerations (7)

The vascularization of the brain is essentially centripetal. The brain i enveloped by a network of leptomeningeal arteries, coming from afferent trunk which remain basal or on the outside. The intracerebral arteries originate fr this peripheral network and converge centripetally towards the ventricles. Th can be classified in cortical, medullary and striate branches, supplying the cortex, the white matter, the grey nuclei and the internal capsule, respectiv In addition, there exists a phylogenetically much older second vascular suppl of centrifugal direction. It orginates from subependymal arteries, which are terminal branches of the choroideal arteries and of certain rami striati laterales, and it supplies the periventricular layers of the brain. There are and this is important to emphasize, no anastomoses between the periventricula centrifugal and the peripheral-centripetal cerebral-vascular supply.

Anastomoses, collateral circulation

Circle of Willis: The are many variations of the circle varying from a completely open ring system of basal vessels to virtually non existing commun cating arteries in the shape of thin threads. Hemodynamic shifts occur if the is adequate lumen of the vessel needed to compensate for a defect of supply b increased flow, e. g. to fill the posterior cerebral artery via the posterior communicating artery.

Heubner's meningeal anastomoses. If the meningeal anastomoses are not narrowed by arteriosclerotic fibrosis (rather than stenosis), they are still likely to act as functional stenosis (in hemodynamic sense), when vessels like the major branches of the middle cerebral artery are to be filled by the retrograde route via meningeal anastomoses with a diameter of less than 0,5 to ·
1,0 mm, for instance, from the anterior cerebral artery.
Neurosurgical experience is such that meningial anastomoses can provide adequate supply in emergencies.

by Schmidt, 1955, does not provide hemodynamically sufficient compensation in infarcts (with sudden onset of collateral demand), but it does so in slowly developing obliterative thrombangitis, where the dilated arachnoid anastomosing vessels cause the impression of macroscopic "hyperemia" (8).

Capillary anastomoses between cortical and striate branches of the peripheral-centripetal cerebrovascular supply do not have sufficient compensatory capacity to prevent the development of an infarct but may serve as sources of reparative processes particularly in infarcts of the "deep" basal ganglia in the region region of the border zone with the "cortical" supply.

Extra-intracranial anastomoses: There are well known anastomoses via the ophthalmic artery (from the external carotid artery via facial artery or an ethmoidal artery), and there are communications between both carotids and between the external carotid and the vertebral arteries as well.

Metahemokinesis (blood diversion)

This phenomenon consists of the diversion of blood from a region or source of vascular supply into an area of demand not normally supplied by this source. It is commonly called "vascular steal". It is caused by demand in an area which cannot be fulfilled because of insufficiency, obstruction or stenosis of the vessel normally supplying this region. Metahemokinesis has been observed in cerebro vascular occlusions, vascular malformations and brain tumors. Patterns of metahemokinesis have been described for the extracranial, intracranial and intracerebral circulation. Willisian metahemokinesis is due to occlusion of one or both carotid arteries. Leptomeningeal metahemokinesis is due to occlusion of the one or both of the anterior, middle vertebral arteries or of the basiliar artery.

A somewhat different cause for intracerebral metahemokinesis has been postulated by Fazio (9): A region is thought to be affected by primary impair-

ment of vasomotor regulation; a neighbouring region supplied by the same art
opens up its collaterals because of increased local demand. Perfusion press
is thought to drop in the region of vasomotor dysfunction, thereby causing
regional ischamia due to metahemokinesis.

The hemodynamic consequences of metahemokinesis may be regional ischemi
in the area from which blood is diverted into the region of demand. In cases
vascular malformation the gradual increase of demand causes initially wideni
of the arteries supplying the angioma. In late stages focal ischemia appears
an area topographically unrelated to the site of the angioma when the blood
demand is so huge that significant diversion of blood occurs.

Regional vasomotor paralysis is a different phenomenon, which may mimic
intracerebral metahemokinesis. Regardless of its cause, it is characterized]
a lack of vasoconstriction during hyperventilation or of vasodilation follow:
inhalation of 5% CO_2. Likewise there is regionally increased flow in a dysau
regulated area when blood pressure is raised from 90 to 130 mm Hg, a measure
which does not increase blood flow in patients or subjects with normal cereb:
autoregulation. Regional vasomotor paralysis therefore is characterized by l
of carbon dioxyde reactivity and loss of autoregulation confined to a circum-
scribed area.

The hemodynamic effects of local vasomotor paralysis are the following:
The vessels are relatively dilated and resistance to perfusion is low. Follo
hyperventilation there will be a general constriction of blood vessels and tl
affected region will appear "hyperemic". Following 5% CO_2 inhalation or phar
cologically induced vasodilatation there will be no vascular response within
affected region which then appears as a zone with relatively low (:ischemic"`
blood flow, or CBF might even further decrease. This has been termed "intracerebral vascular steal"

There are two explanations for this phenomenon: One, the cerebral vesse:
are fixed at an intermediate diameter during vasomotor paralysis and act lik
rigid tubes. Therefore blood flow remains very much the same at rest and dur:
general vasodilatation by 5% CO_2 inhalation. Since they are paralyzed at an
intermediate level of widening they cannot react to CO_2. Therefore they perm:
passive blood flow to the same extent as during rest. The other explanatio
advanced by Lassen (10) is based on the bservation of a distinct, absolute
decrease of regional blood flow in the affected region, i.e. lower CBF value:
during CO_2 inhalation compared to the values in the same region at rest (not
only lower than the rest of the brain). This is thought to be the consequenc

of passive compression of the vasoparalytic vessels due to the increase in the intracranial pressure provoked by the 5% CO_2 inhalation.

In a study of 52 apoplexies, Lassen and Skinhøj (10) observed a dissociation of the regional extent of those responses. While lack of CO_2 reactivity was confined to the affected region, autoregulation was lost in the entire hemisphere. In 21 tumor cases the same authors report hemispheric loss of autoregulation on the ipsilateral side of the tumor, i. e. no vasoconstriction following induced hypertension. On the other hand CO_2 reactivity remained normal, indicating vasoconstriction in the entire hemisphere.

Regions of supernormal ("hyperemic") flow can be identified in acute apoplexy using Xenon-133 regional quantitative cerebral blood flow measurements. This regional hyperemia is seen at the periphery of the ischemic lesion or even covering the entire lesion. It is a transitory phenomenon lasting only a few hours or a few days at the most (11).

This focal hyperfusion may also be seen by angiography (12). The angiographic findings are characterized by an early filling of the veins with contrast media draining the affected region.

Another finding was a "blush" in the region drained by the veins filling early; occasionally this blush was the only sign of the regional cerebrovascular abnormality. When studied by the 133-Xe method the same region revealed exceptionally rapid perfusion (12).

Focal impairment of regional cerebral blood flow

Focal reduction of cerebral blood flow can be observed in transistory ischemic attacks (TIA), prolonged reversible ischemic attacks, or in completed strokes.

The causes of focal reduction of CBF are

1. Arterial stenoses or
2. Obstructions due to in situ thrombosis from atheroma or arteritis
3. Obstructions due to emboli
4. Intracerebral steal (metahemokinesis)
5. Vasospasm by hemodynamic dysfuction

TIA and prolonged reversible ischemic attacks

A multifactor genesis is considered (13) including disturbances of the microcirculation. It is thought that there is a region of vasomotor paralysis with disturbed functional metabolism due to an episode of oxygen deficiency. Structural metabolism is thought to be unaltered, however, recently evidence cerebral infarcts displayed by CT has been reported in 18 - 79% (14).

Cerebral infarcts

Occlusion of major vessel frequently results in cerebral infarction whic is characterized by a necrotization and softening of the neural tissue. Occlu sion may be caused by embolism, thrombosis or angiopathy.
Encephalomalacia may also be caused by hemodynamic dysfunction without arteri obstruction or stenosis. On the other hand gradual occlusion of a cerebral ar tery does not necessarily produce cerebral infarction. When the brain is thre ened by ischemia resulting fron vascular obstruction or stenosis, the fixed collaterals must be utilized for adequate blood flow through the threatened region. If these collaterals are adequate and if blood flow can be restored infarction may not occur; if collateral stimulation is inadequate for any rea the regional lack of oxygen causes infarct necrosis. Encephalomalacias may be white or red. Red brain softenings are hemorrhagic infarcts with incomplete necrosis of tissue, distension of the capillaries and venules and pericapilla erythrodiapedesis,predominantly in cortex or basal ganglia. These morpholo- gical findings may explain the observations of "early filling of veins"(12) in carotid angiography or the "regional hyperfusion" (11) in apoplexy in Xeno 133 regional CBF estimations. Cerebral infarcts can be visualized on static radionuclide imaging of the brain with variable intensity of uptake between hours after the apoplexy to several months later.

"Luxury perfusion" syndrome

It may be defined as dissociation of local blood flow and local metabol Hypoglycemia causes reduction of tissue pCO_2, due to depressed glucose metabol Both CBF and cerebral tissue pO_2 decrease, render the brain more susceptible the effects of hyperventilation since the decrease òf blood flow further limi the available glucose. Oxygen availability to the tissue is also reduced. Injection of glucose during hypoglycenia rapidly brings about an increased cortical pCO_2 indicating that an increase in cerebral metabolism brought about by restoration of deficient substrate increases CBF.This observation makes it clear that cerebral blood flow follows tissue demands.

When cerebral hypoxia is induced in cats,by temporary exsanguination followed by resanguination,continuing depression of the EEG (low frequencies) can be observed while blood flow measurements show markedly increased flow. This observation is a clear hint that cerebral flow can be increased without correspondingly increased levels of tissue metabolism.

When 15-O_2 first came into use brain oxygen consumption was determined and also regional dissociation was found between oxygen supply and metabolism as an expression of seeming dissociation of blood flow and cerebral metabolism.

In patients with acute vascular lesions Ingvar (11) observed foci of profound EEG slowing associated with increased or normal blood flow. More recently, Kuhl's group demonstrated regional depression of cerebral metabolism in a region with diminished 18-Fluoro deoxyglucose uptake associated with disproportionally higher blood flow shown in the same region by local depositon of B-NH_3. The method of visualization was positron emission computer tomography (PET). The subject was a patient with non-hemorragic stroke with right homonymous hemianopsia and alexia who was studied 8 days after the onset of his cerebrovascular insult (15).

It is not known presently if blood flow through an area of the brain damaged by regional anoxia is maintained because of incomplete obstruction of the artery supplying the affected region or by intracerebral diversion of blood flow from neighbouring regions via anastomoses. Both may be the case, but it is difficult to know in the individual patient. This type of regional blood flow has been termed "luxury perfusion". It is maintained for a short time only, after which it ceases. If local metabolic need (tissue demand) is considered the principal intrinsic cerebral determinant of regional alterations of cerebral blood flow, then luxury perfusion would be a logical consequence after an episode of ischemia without being luxurious at all. In this sense postischemic, reactive hyperfusion is a necrosity in order to attempt as much tissue oxygenation and restitution as possible. Since CO_2 reactivity and autoregulation are lost in regional post ischemic perfusion, this phenomenon must be looked upon as vasomotor paralysis (dilatation) of the vessels permitting passive perfusion rather than as a form of active hyperemia. From a teleological point of view regional post ischemic perfusion serves as the optimum attempt for restitution of anoxic or hypoxic cerebral tissue damage. With respect to the pathogenesis of episodes of regional ischemia the effectiveness of the autonomous nervous

system to change the fractional distribution of cardiac output as well as to
initiate compensatory responses in the cerebral vascular bed remains unsolved.

Investigation methods and nuclides

From the viewpoint of radiopharmacology it becomes apparent that there is
a clinical need for radionuclide studies in patients in order to elucidate
cerebrovascular insufficiency. In particular, measurements are required to
localize and quantify the extent of metabolic depression of regional tissue
damage after an episode of ischemia, to follow changes in regional metabolic
activity during the course of therapy, and finally to follow changes in region
blood flow inclusive of assessment of regional CO_2 reactivity and autoregulati

From the viewpoint of the radionuclide methods used it is evident that al
techniques based on transit time alone will fail to make a correct quantitativ
assessment of blood flow. The observation of postischemic regional perfusion
("luxury perfusion") using the Xenon-133 regional CBF assessment makes it clea
that a different tracer is needed to demonstrate postischemic tissue damage.
Deoxyglucose, of course is such a tracer, and may be labelled with Carbon-11
or Fluor-18. These ultra shortliving positron emitters (20 min and 100 min) mu
be produced by a cyclotron locally at a minimum starting investment of
approximately 1.000.000,-- US $ each for the building, the cyclotron and the
positron emission computer tomography instrument; annual operating costs are
estimated at 200.000,-- US $ at the present time. It can be safely assumed tha
only a few large medical centers will be equipped to perform PECT studies in
the future. Radiopharmacological research, of course, will be stimulated by th
need of simultaneous visualization and quantification of regional cerebral
metabolism and blood flow. New tracers to study cerebral blood flow will be
Kr-81m dissolved in saline, and Tantalum-178 obtained from Wolfram-178 generators. Whether or not J-123-Isopropyl-amphetamine resembles Deoxyglucose in its
proportionality of uptake to metabolic activity remains to be seen.

The property of 99m-Tc-chelates to show nonseptic damage of the blood
brain barrier in static radionuclide imaging of the brain will probably retain
its clinical usefullness, particulary in the demonstration of absence of localized tissue damage after transient or protracted ischemis attacks.

Sequential imaging of the first pass of a non diffusible tracer througt
the cranio-cerebral circulation should have a role in the assessmant of the
functional effectiveness of vascular necrosis. It is a method which is able to
visualize reiably the unilateral delay of cerebral perfusion in relatively

large infarcts in the middle cerebral artery distribution. It remains to be seen how effectively it can demonstrate areas of postischemic perfusion, or vasomotor paralysis, respectively.

REFERENCES

1. Jones CE: Control of cardiac output. Cardiovascular flow dynamics and measurements, Hwang NHC, Normann NA (eds), Baltimore, University Park Pre 1977, p 365-401.

2. Ott E: Einfluss eines zentralen cholinergen Wirkungsmechanisnmus auf die Regulation der intakten und gestörten zerebralen Durchblutung. Fortschr. Neurol.Psychait.8: 452-468, 1978.

3. Shalit MN, Reinmuth O, Shimojyo S, Scheinberg P: A mechanism by which car dioxide influences cerebral circulation independent of a direct effect on vascular smooth muscle. Research on the cerebral circulation, Third Inter national Salzburg Conference, Meyer JS, Lechner H, Eichhorn O (eds), Springfield, Charles C. Thomas, 1969, p 173-185.

4. Kety S: Possible applications of regional blood flow measured by autoradi graphic techniques. In: Research on the cerebral circulation, Third Inter national Salzburg Conference, Meyer JS, Lechner H, Eichhorn O, (eds), Springfield, Charles C. Thomas, 1969, p 83-85.

5. Fieschi C: Cerebral blood flow in neurological and neurosurgical patients Radionuclide applications in neurology and neurosurgery, Wang Y, Paoletti P (eds), Springfield, Charles C Thomas, 1970, p 55-75.

6. Meyer JS, Welch KMA: Relationships of cerebral blood flos and metabolism neurological symptoms. Progress in brain research 12, Meyer JS, Schade JP (eds), Amsterdam, Elsevier, 1972.

7. Van den Bergh R: The periventricular intracerebral blood supply. Research on the cerebral circulation, Fourth International Salzburg Conference, Meyer JS, Reivich M, Lechner H, Eichhorn O (eds), Springfield, Charles C Thomas, 1970, p 52-65.

8. Zülch KJ, Kleihues P, Gabe D: Die aktuelle Problematik auf dem Gebiet der Pathogenese, Klinik und Therapie der Hirndurchblutungsstörungen. Der Hirnkreislauf in Forschung und Klinik, Kongressband des II. Salzburger Symposions, Wien, Hollinik, 1964, p 339-364.

9. Fazio C: The importance of the "Intracerebral Steal" in the pathogenesis of focal brain ischemia. Research on the cerebral circulation, Fourt Inte national Salzburg Conference, Meyer JS, Reivich M, Lechner H, Eichhorn O (eds), Springfield, Charles C Thomas, 1970, p 57-59.

10. Lassen NA, Skinhøj E: Regional cerebral blood flow measurements disclosin abnormally perfused tissue somponents and "Intracerebral Steal" in cases apoplexy and brain tumors. Research on the cerebral circulation, Fourth International Salzburg Conference, Meyer JS, Reivich M, Lechner H, Eichho ¼ (eds), Springfield, Charles C Thomas, 1970, p 76-79.

11. Lassen NA, Ingvar DH: Regional cerebral blood flow in apoplexy: studies o its pathophysiology, using 8 to 16 external detectors with the Xenon 133 method. Research on the cerebral circulation, Third International Confere Meyer JS, Lechner H, Eichhorn O (eds), Springfield, Charles C Thomas, 196 p 96-107.

12. Cronqvist S: Transistory hyperemia in focal cerebral ischemic lesions. Research on the cerebral circulation, Third International Salzburg Conference, Meyer JS, Lechner H, Eichhorn O (eds), Springfield, Charles C Thomas, 1969, p 71-82.

13. Lechner H, Ladurner G, Ott E: Die zerebralen transistorisch ischaemischen Attacken, Hans Huber, Bern, 1979.

14. Ladurner G, Sager WD, Iliff CD, Lechner H: A correlation of clinical findings and CT in ischemic cerebrovascular disease. Eur Neurol 18: 281-288, 1979.

15. Hawkins RA, Phelps ME, Huang SC, Kuhl DE: Effect of ischemia on quantification of local cerebral glucose metabolic rate in man. Journal of Cerebral Blood Flow and Metabolism 1: 37-51, 1981.

TECHNETIUM REAGENTS FOR CEREBRAL IMAGING: A REVIEW

C. APRILE

INTRODUCTION

Rapid advances in the technology of Single Photon Emission Computed Tomography (SPECT) have renewed the interest of clinicians and radiopharmacologists in the field of nuclear neurology as far as better spatial resolution and the possibility to obtain quantitative functional images are concerned.

The last point especially has led to the selection of single photon emitting nuclides for in vivo tracer studies, with reference to: physical half-life matched with the time of the study, high yield of nuclear events able to provide a high count rate for reconstruction algorithms, low dose to the patient and the possibility of labelling various chemical substrates with high specific activity. In this respect Atkins and coworkers (1) have recently calculated the figure of merit of single photon nuclides according to the formula:

$$\text{figure of Merit (photons/rad)} = \frac{\text{photons/uCi} \times e^{-\lambda t} \times G \times P}{\text{rad/uCi} \times h \times \tau}$$

where G is the geometrical plane source efficiency, P is the crystal photopeak efficiency and τ is the average life. Altough this formula serves only as a general guide from the physical point of view and does not take into account specific localization in target organs, Tc^{99m} appears to be the choice nuclide for SPECT at a time interval of up to 4 hours, followed by ^{123}I.

Until recently, labelled reagents suitable for brain imaging could be divided into the following four categories:

1. Radiopharmaceuticals (RP) capable of crossing through "disrupted" Blood Brain Barrier (BBB) and concentrating in space occupying lesions.
2. Agents remaining in the vascular space and measuring Cerebral Blood Volume.
3. Agents suitable for regional Cerebral Blood Flow measure.
4. RP capable of crossing intact BBB.

172

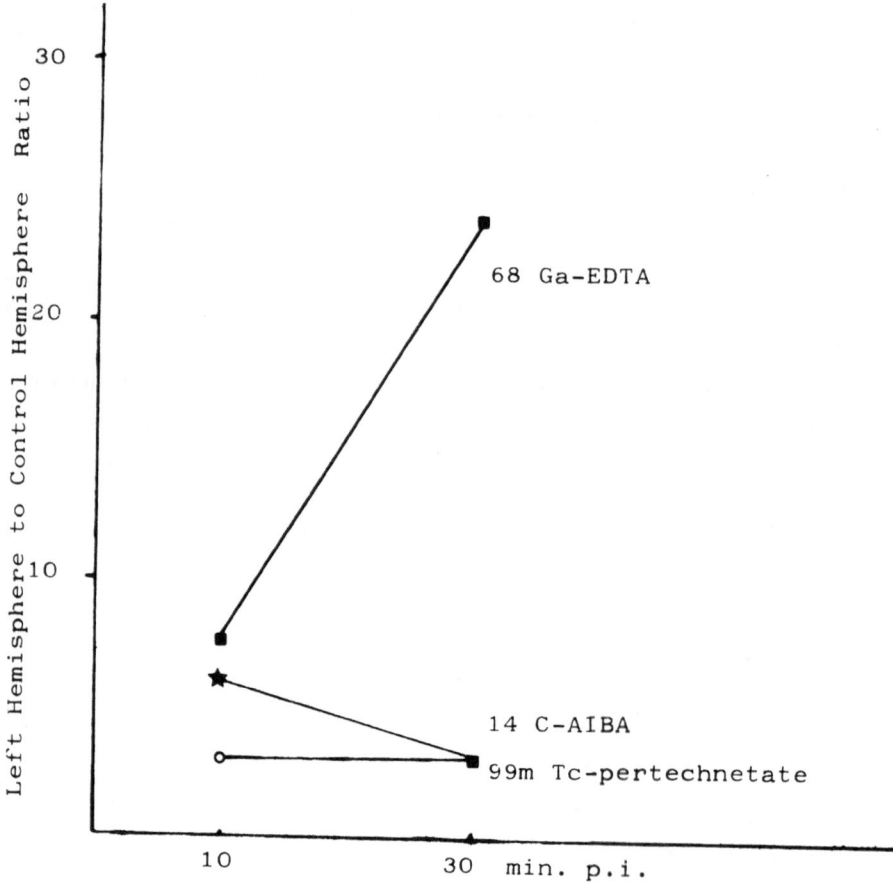

Fig. 1. Left hemisphere to control rats hemisphere ratio, after monolateral disruption, 10 and 30 min post injection of 68 Ga-EDTA, 11 C-aminoisobutyric acid and Tc[99m] pertechnetate. (data from ref. 3).

Tc-labelled reagents demonstrating disruption of the Blood Brain Barrie

'Although uncertainties exist about where BBB has an anatomical location, has been demonstrated (2) that tumours with open endothelial junctions (widt 75-200 Å) accumulate pertechnetate to a high degree while tight junctions ar associated with reduced uptake of the tracer. In other words, the suitabilit a RP is related to the ability to distinguishing a BBB lesion in a backgrour normal brain. In this connection using an experimental rat model to obtain F disruption after hyperosmolar mannitol infusion into the left carotid artery Washburn and coworkers (3) measured the uptake of $Tc^{99m} O_4$, 14 C-AIBA and 68 Ga-EDTA at 10 and 30 min after intravenous injection (fig. 1). The results

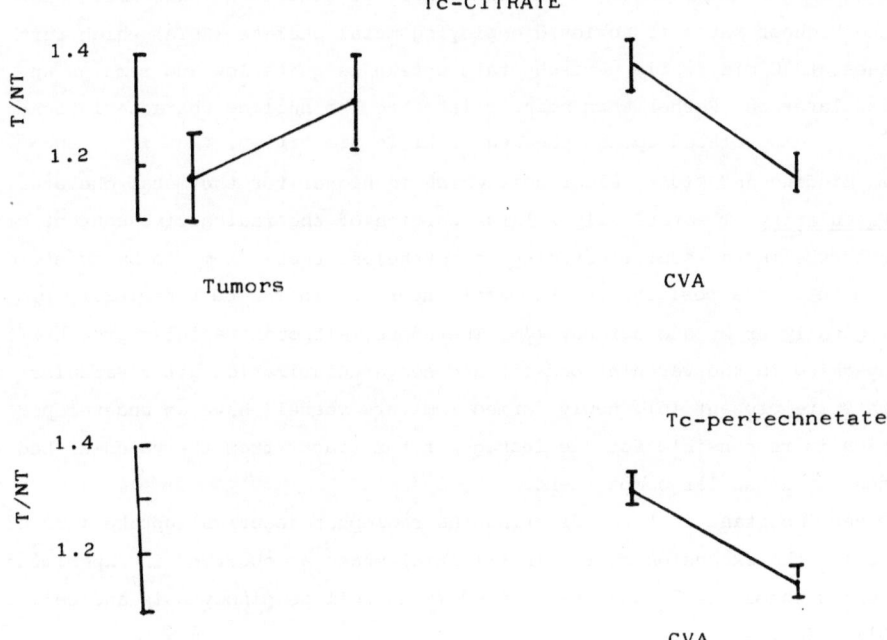

Fig. 2. Values of the T/NT ratio 30 and 360 min post injection in cerebrovascular accidents (CVA) and tumours. Difference between citrate en pertechnetate (Paired Student's t-test) is not significant.

Table I

Evaluation of Tc^{99m}-glucoheptonate as brain scanning agent	
(early and late scan)	
Overall sensitivity	83%
(CVA	62%)
(Tumours	94%)
Accuracy	95.5%
	(Tanasescu et al. 1977)

expressed as Left Hemisphere to the Hemisphere of Control animals Ratio show
that the highest ratio is achieved employing metal chelate (EDTA) which furth
increases at 30 min, while pertechnetate uptake is quite low and remains unmodified later on. Rather than being related to the nuclide characteristics,
such data seems related to the chemical vehicle properties, that is to the
protein binding and kidney clearance, which is higher for the metal chelates.

Vascularity. Theoretically a large portion of the radioactive content ca
be due to the intravascular activity; nevertheless there seems to be no stric
relation between a positive pertechnetate scan and increased vascularity prov
histologically or by angiography (4). Therefore, although vascular growth wit
cells packing in the vascular bed (5) and neovascularization after vascular
accidents are present (6), newly formed immature vessels have an undeveloped
BBB which is responsible for the leakage of the tracer from the vascular bed
into the extravascular compartment.

Other important factors affecting the radiopharmaceutical uptake into br
lesions are the expansion of the interstitial space as observed in experiment
mouse brain tumour (4,7) and reactive edema as well as pinocytosis and cellul
metabolism (8).

Pertechnetate, Tc-chelates and Tc-bone seekers

After its introduction into nuclear medicine practice Tc^{99m} pertechnetat
was the agent of choice for brain scanning: later a group of other Tc-complex
have been introduced such as DTPA (9), citrate (10), glucoheptonate (GH) (11)
and gluconate (GA) (12). Common characteristics of such Tc-compounds are:
negative electrical charge, fast blood-clearance via the kidney, low serum
protein binding, absent uptake by the thyroid, salivary glands, choroid plexu
and gastric mucosa and significant uptake in kidney cortex except for DTPA wh
is excreted by glomular filtration. In addition Tc-labelled bone seekers have
been proposed in the detection of vascular brain accidents (13). From the clii
al point of view, these compounds have been intensively studied and a large
number of articles have been published, related to the following points:
- Overall sensitivity of Tc-chelates vs. pertechnetate.
- Specificity in discriminating neoplastic from vascular lesions.
- Detectability of the lesions during early and delayed scan.
- Differential diagnosis between lesions located in the skull, meninges or in
  the brain itself.
Although the reported data are not immediately comparable, because of differer

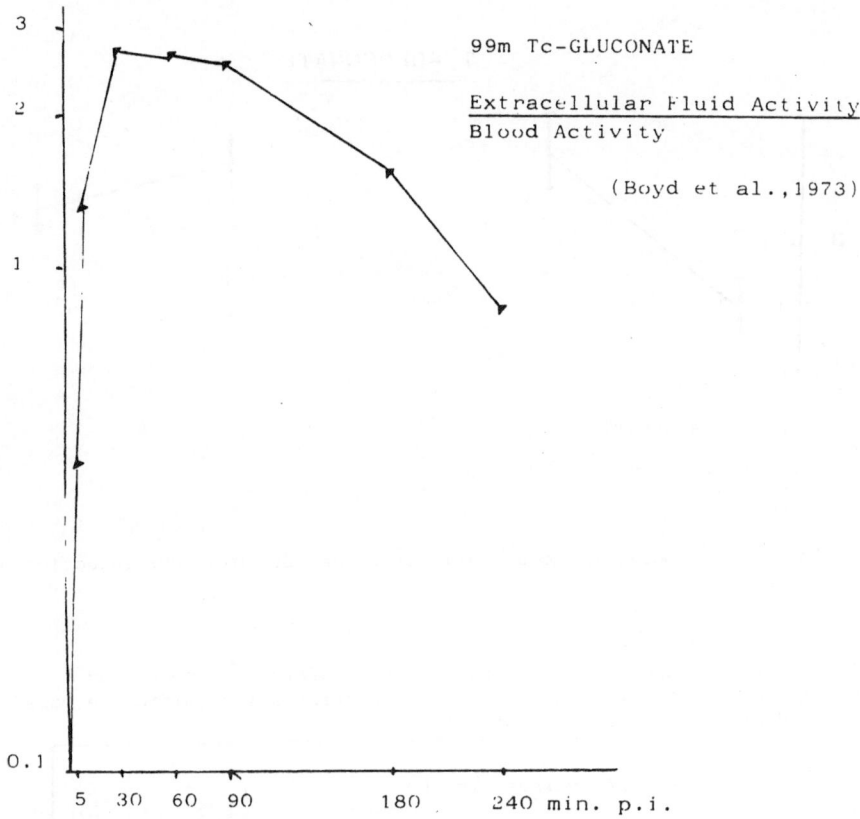

Fig. 3. Data from ref. 24.

techniques used in recording data and different criteria for the evaluation of
scans, some conclusions can be drawn.

Citrate versus pertechnetate

In the case of vascular accidents slightly better results were achieved
with citrate only in terms of the definition of normal anatomy as well as regions
of abnormal uptake, while the tumour/non tumour ratio decreases from the early
(30 min) to the late scan (6 hours post injection) or remains unchanged as with
citrate or pertechnetate (14) (fig. 2). Brain tumours both primary and metastatic were better visualized with citrate, the tumour/non tumour ratio rising
significantly between the late scans, while pertechnetate shows only a slight
increase (15). This different behaviour of pertechnetate and citrate has also
been described by others (16,17).

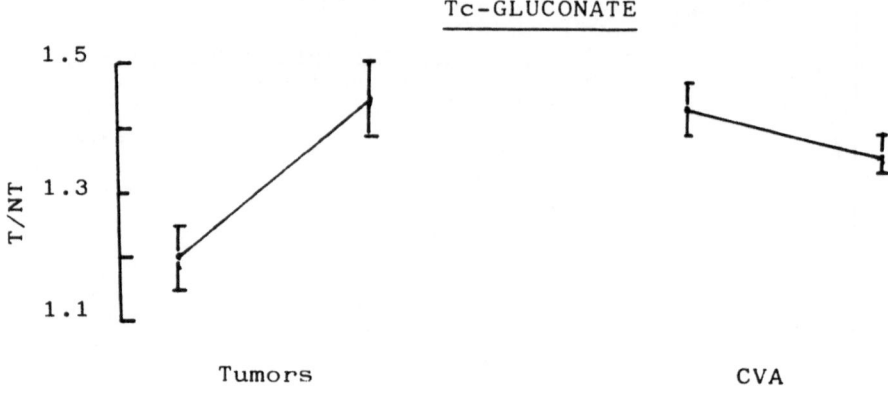

Fig. 4. Values of tumour/non tumour ratio at 30 and 360 min post injection o
Tc-gluconate.

Table II. Lesion to background ratio in cerebral infarcts, tumours and
metastases 180 min post injection of Tc-DTPA. Statistical significance based
on paired Student's t-test. Data from ref. 28.

	Tc-DTPA versus Tc-PPi		
	Lesion to background ratio		
	Cerebral Infarcts	Tumours (primary)	Tumours (metastases)
DTPA	1.55	2.41	1.66
PPi	1.42	1.21	1.23
	p n.s.	p<.05	p<.05
			(Kim, 1980)

Glucoheptonate and DTPA versus pertechnetate

Similar results in terms of the definition of normal anatomy, abnormal
uptake and higher lesion to non-lesion ratio were reported in the series of
Rollo and coworkers (18) and by the Los Angeles group (11, 19, 20, 21) when
comparing the behaviour of the three tracers. GH appears to concentrate in al:
lesions which accumulate DTPA and pertechnetate and, in certain cases, it

showed lesions missed by the two other tracers, although generally Tumour/non tumour ratios are about equal with DTPA and GH on visual inspection. In addition, these authors did not find any significant pattern of variation of the tumour/ non tumour ratio in neoplastic or vascular diseases. An early scan at 30 min post injection may miss a significant number of lesions while the 90 and 180 min scans provide the same diagnostic accuracy (table I). Computing the Calvaria / Brain ratio at 30 min post injection Rollo found an average value of 1.6 for TcO_4 and 2.1 for Tc-GH, indicating an increased background level for pertechnetate with an associated low tumour / not tumour ratio. On the other hand Leveille et al (22) found that GH was a superior reagent for the detection of brain tumours, but this is not entirely true for cerebral infarctions.

Gluconate

Tc-gluconate like other Tc-chelates, shows a very fast blood-clearance via the kidney (23) with a maximum Extracellular Fluid/Blood Ratio at 30 min post injection (24) (fig. 3), which decreases with time suggesting that extra- cellular fluid pool constitutes a compartment quickly filled by Tc-GA. After it releases the RP back to the blood-pool to maintain an equilibrium between the two compartments. In fig. 4 the time course of the tumour/non tumour ratio from early to late scan is shown, with a decrease or with no change at all in vascular lesions, while in neoplastic diseases the ratio tends to rise with time. In contrast to citrate, tumour/non tumour values achieved with Tc-GA either in the early or in the late scan are generally higher that with TcO_4, also in the case of vascular diseases (25,16). When comparing the accuracy of GA, citrate, pertechnetate and DTPA in the detection of brain tumours Ackerman and coworkers (26) found GA to be superior to pertechnetate and citrate, and nearly equal to DTPA.

Tc-phosphate compounds

Tc-phosphate complexes have been reported by various authors (13,27) to concentrate in vascular diseases of the brain, allowing differential diagnosis from tumours, which do not take up the RP in significant amounts. Although differential diagnosis was achieved by the above authors employing pertechnetate and phosphate compounds, Kin and coworkers (28) studying patients with brain lesions with DTPA and PPi showed no significant differences in the Target to Background Ratio as far as cerebral infarcts are concerned, while in neoplastic diseases, Tc-DTPA was far superior to PPi (table II).

178

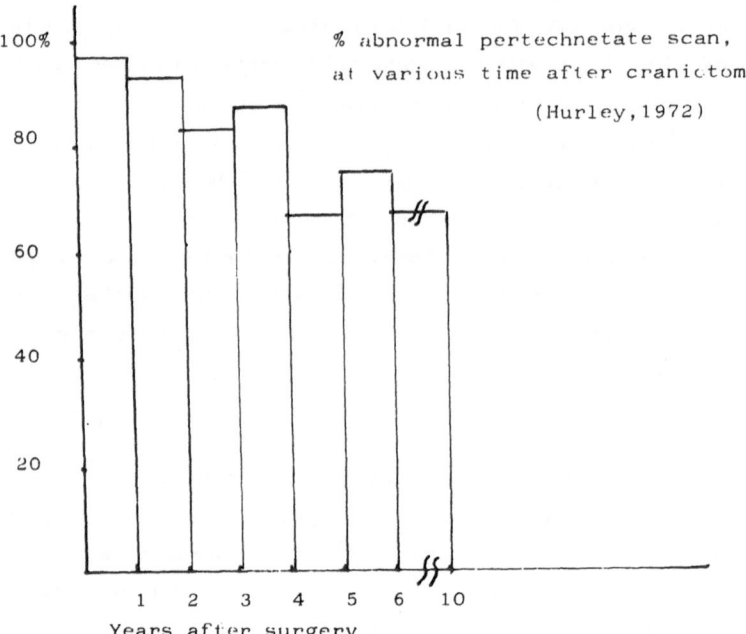

Fig. 5. Data from ref. 32.

Tc-bleomycin

Efforts to label bleomycin (BLM) with Tc^{99m} are aimed at combining the
specificity of the antibiotic compound with the favourable physical characteri
tics of Tc^{99m}. Unfortunately unsuccessful tumour scanning with Tc-BLM has been
reported (29), indicating that labelling with nuclides different from Co or Cu
alters the chemical properties and metabolism of the compound. Accumulation of
Tc-BLM to some extent into brain neoplasms has only been reported by a Japanes
group (30,31) who observed a higher detection rate for glioma, meningioma and
metastatic tumours, slightly superior to that of pertechnetate (65% vs 60%). I
a comparative study, Tc-GA was proven to be superior to Tc-BLM in the detectio
of brain metastases (26).

Postcraniotomy

It is well known that surgical lesions of the skull can result in long
standing abnormalities on brain scans (fig. 5), possibly due to a prolonged ab
normality in the skeletal extracellular fluid space (32). Generally a multi-
nuclide approach has been proposed employing Ga^{67}-citrate, pertechnetate and T

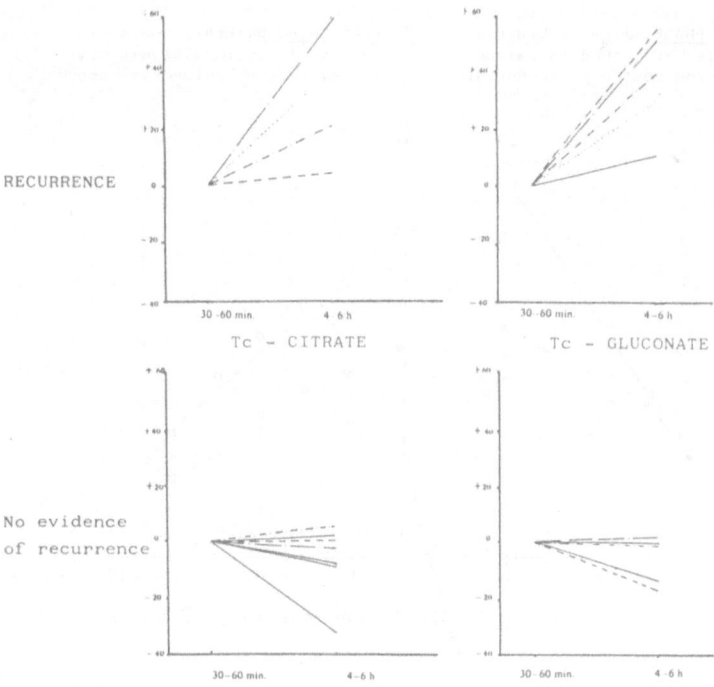

Fig. 6. Percent variation of the T/NT ratio in patients previously submitted to surgery for brain tumours after injection of Tc-citrate and Tc-gluconate.

phosphate compound (33), based on the fact that Ga-uptake did not occur when tumour recurrence is not present, although presence of inflammation or infections of the surgical flap would preclude this evaluation. In order to simplify the nuclide approach Hill et al. (34) proposed the comparison of the one hour and two hours scan after injection of Tc-DTPA. A definite increase in intensity is observed when tumour recurrence is present. Evaluation of the T/NT ratio % variation between early and late scan employing citrate of gluconate was proposed (14,25). We observed a significant increase of the ratio when tumour recurrence was present. Similar results were obtained with both tracers although the accuracy was slightly better when using Tc-GA. (fig. 6).

Discussion

A major drawback of the Tc-compounds which have been discussed is their poor specificity, although the study of the wash-out rate from the lesion can help in differentiating vascular from neoplastic aetiology. Furthermore their exact mechanism of action has been elucidated to a relatively lesser degree when

180

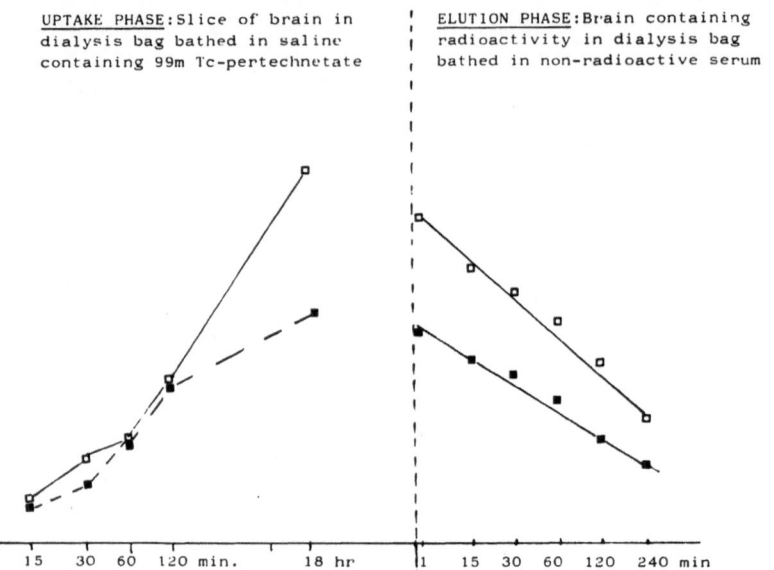

UPTAKE PHASE:Slice of brain in
dialysis bag bathed in saline
containing 99m Tc-pertechnetate

ELUTION PHASE:Brain containing
radioactivity in dialysis bag
bathed in non-radioactive serum

| 15 30 60 120 min. | 18 hr | 1 15 30 60 120 240 min |

Fig. 7. Affinity of brain tissue for pertechnetate (data from ref. 35).

compared, for instance, to the infarct avid tracers employed in nuclear cardiol-
ogy. In this regard, the following points, in addition to the disruption of BBB
must be considered in order to elucidate the behaviour of the compounds in
normal and pathological brain.

- Binding to the macromolecules in the interstitial fluid.
- Cellular membrane binding.
- Passage through altered cellular membrane.
- Intracellular binding.

    It is well known that pertechnetate is virtually excluded from brain tissu
even when the tissue is a post-mortem specimen, in which BBB mechanisms are not
functioning (35). (Fig. 7). Since proteins are present in the vascular, intracellular and intracellular space, knowledge of the Affinity Constant (AC) of Tc
compounds may provide information about the mechanism of localization. Albumin
the most important protein present in the vascular and interstitial space; at p
7.4 it is above the isoelectric point of 5.5 and contains about 100 positively
charged and 100 negatively charged sites, each or a combination of them able to
bind charged molecules, but the anion binding is prevalent to the cation bindir
Dewanjee recently reported (36) the AC of some metal chelates for albumin emplc
ing the Scatchard method: the AC was found to be highest for Tc-DMSA and lowest

Table III. Affinity Constant (AC) for HSA of various Tc-compounds
(Data from ref. 36)

	DMSA	PPi	GH	DTPA	TcO_4
LAC x 10^3	22.8	5.5	6.3	1.8	1.9
HAC x 10^5	1.2	0.9	1.1	0.5	–

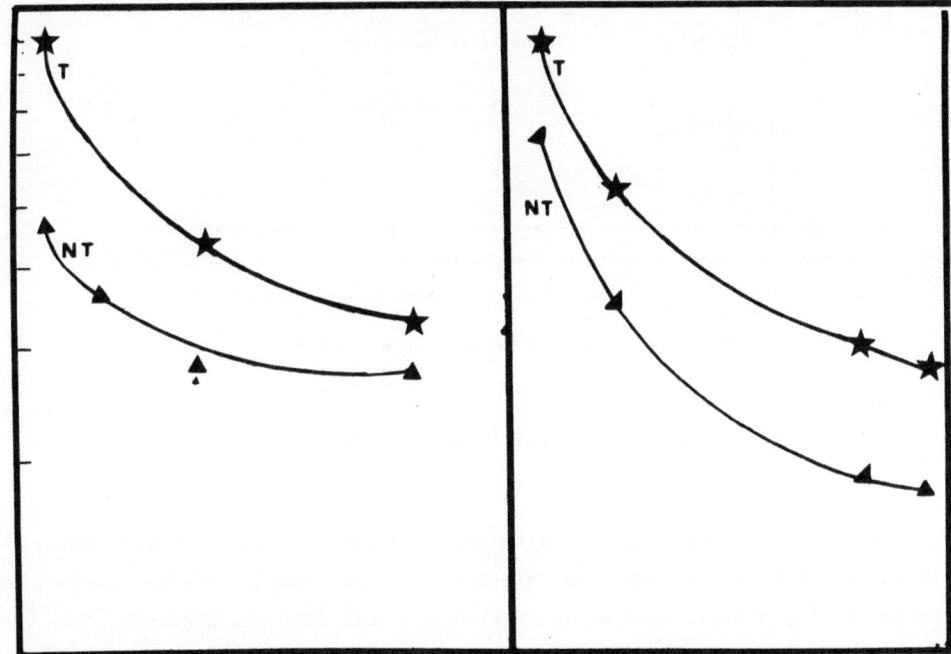

Fig. 8. Time course activity of Tc-gluconate in human pathological tissues.
T: Target. NT: Non Target tissue. Left: inflammatory lesion, Right: tumour.

Table IV. Tc^{99m}-gluconate uptake in mice melanoma (Hunt, 1980)

hours p.i.	% i.d. / g	tumour/muscle ratio
2	1.7	5.3
24	0.5	11.7

182

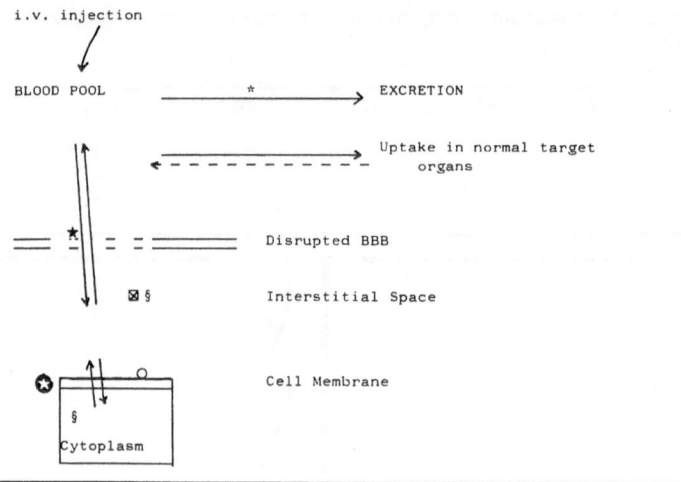

* Binding to plasmatic protein can affect excretion

Chemical structure of the compound can affect ★the passage throuh
disrupted BBB and ☒ AC for protein

§ Denaturation of soluble proteins and pH shift can increase AC

O Hypothetic

✪ M.W. and net electrical charge

Fig. 9. Rate of Tc-compounds in brain lesions after i.v. injection and factor
affecting their distribution.

for Tc-DTPA (Table III). Binding with pertechnetate is very weak and easily d
placed by a variety of competing molecules (35) presumably because it binds o
one positively charged site while Tc-chelates form multiple bindings. This
behaviour is very similar to that observed with BSA, β and γ globulin. Poor
protein binders distribute immediately after i.v. injection into the ECF and
quickly excreted by GF, while other chelates bound to HSA to a higher degree
distribute more slowly, but have more time to be absorbed in target organs. W
blood-levels decrease, RP with high AC will be retained in the target for a
longer time.

    In addition to an expanded protein pool in the interstitial space, other
factors can increase AC:
- Denaturation of soluble proteins, for instance it has been demonstrated tha
  Tc-MDP has a higher affinity for heat denatured than for negative HSA (37).
- pH shift: at a low pH most of the proteic macromolecules remain in the dena
  ated state, enhancing non specific binding. In other words the retention ti
  in pathological tissue will be increased with higher Lesion/Background rati

In no case was real permanent accumulation of such a compound into pathological cells observed (38). On the other hand we have demonstrated that human viable lymphocytes, when incubated in Hank's solution, show a binding of Tc-GA, not removable by dilution of the medium, but markedly decreased by brief trypsinization. In addition, this binding is not demonstrable when cells are incubated in plasma (39). These results are consistent with the hypothesis that Tc-GA potentially binds to cellular membrane ligands of normal cells, but the presence of plasma inhibits this attachment, either by competitive binding or saturation of cellular membrane ligands.

In the presence of altered membrane permeability as in tumours, diffusion of ionic non specific RP can be enhanced (38) according to the Cox and Van der Pompe model, in which the uptake into the cells is not specific, related to the cell membrane permeability, according to the Nerst equation and influenced by the electrical charge and the molecular weight (40,42).

After heat killing (56°C per one hour) the number of non viable lymphocytes increases without reduction of the cells number, and the cellular uptake of Tc-gluconate is 3-4 times higher than in viable lymphocytes, it means that the tracer can diffuse across altered membrane, in fact the dilution of the incubating medium causes wash-out from the inner cell to the medium (39). The main difference between Tc-compounds and In or Ga-compounds is that there is not an intracellular stable binding, activity in the lesion reaches a maximum and afterwards decreases although the T/NT ratio can increase (40,41,23) (fig. 8 and table IV). This fact does not exclude the possibility that an intracellular binding to normal or denaturated proteins can occur, but it is likely that it is only transient and does not preclude wash-out from the inner cell when relative concentration in the interstitial space and blood-pool decreases.

The tissue and plasma associated factors capable of causing a significant uptake in brain lesions are summarized in fig. 9. The different wash-out rate observed with citrate and gluconate between neoplastic and non-neoplastic lesions, is probably due to the relative abundance of proteic factors and cellular density, capable of prolonging retention time of the RP in the lesion.

Tc-compounds measuring Cerebral Blood Volume

Cerebral Blood Volume (CBV) is an important factor in the control of cerebral hemodynamics. Significant changes are observed during seizure, sleep and mental activity, in infarct tissue (ischemia in and vasodilatation around), after head trauma and cerebral edema. Any Tc-compound which remains in the in the blood-pool for sufficient time, Tc-RBC and at a lesser degree Tc-HSA, can permit measurement of such parameter with the aid of a tomographic system, according to the general formula (43,44,45,46):

$$r\ CBV = \frac{cpm/ml\ in\ ROI}{cpm/ml\ venous\ blood\ x\ 0.85\ x\ d}\ x\ 100$$

where d is the density of cerebral tissue and 0.85 is the correction factor for the difference between large vessels and cerebral hematocrits. In normal subjects, the mean CBV value for the whole brain is 4.34 ml/100 g, while after head trauma the most common pattern is a reduction of about 10% compared to the value after recuperation and greater changes are seen in rCBV.

Tc-compounds measuring cerebral blood-flow

Tc-labelled microspheres after intracarotid injection are trapped in the microvasculature and their distribution is proportional to the regional Cerebral Blood-Flow (rCBF). With Xe CBF is greater in a peripheral band and the region of the Sylvian fissure, whereas with Tc-microsphere, the activity is homogeneously distributed on the external profile, while the pathological patterns are very similar with both tracers (47). The clinical usefulness of this method is limited by the carotid injection, while with Xe CBF evaluation is possible also after intravenous injection or inhalation. With this technique, after surgical STA-MCA (Superficial Tamporary A. - Middle Cerebral A.) anastomosis, it is possible to evaluate (48):
- Patency of the by-pass.
- The area of intracranial vascular filling.
- Changes in the collateral circulation.
The relative advantage over Xe technique is that the latter method does not clearly show the area perfused by the by-pass.

Tc-complexes transported through the blood brain barrier

At present, a limit of SPECT is its low spatial resolution if compared to X-ray CT; therefore there is a major need for a Tc-compound giving more information about metabolic aspects of the brain rather than demonstrating anatomical details. In fact, an agent capable of crossing the intact BBB and of being completely extracted during the first passage may give information about blood-flow which is 400% greater in the grey matter, while the specific gravity is only 0.2% greater in grey than in white matter (49). A substance can be trans-

ported through the BBB and gain access to the extracellular fluid of the CNS by:
- Passive transport, limited to those molecules with a sufficient high Partition
  Coefficient (Olive Oil/Water ≥ 0.03).
- Active transport, which is a carrier mediated system for hydrophilic metabolic
  substances.

The basic requirements for these potential complexes transported by passive
transport are:
- Lipophilicity.
- No functional group with a charge at physiological pH.
- Possibility to be injected intravenously.
- Low serum protein binding.
- Passage through the lung without loss to alveolar air.
- Complete extraction by the brain at the first passage.
- Sufficiently slow wash-out rate from the brain to allow scintigraphic detec-
  tion.

Loberg and coworkers (50) have recently identified three groups of Tc-
complexes which can potentially fulfil the above requirements:
- Tc-complexes with substituted carbamoylmethyliminodiacetates.
- Tc-complexes with substituted aminopolycarboxylates.
- Tc-substituted oxines.
Among these, the H and I oxine substituted molecules appear to be the most
promising agents, with high Octanol/Buffer partition coefficient (23.6% and
78.5%) and high Brain Uptake Index (53.6% and 68.6%) despite a quite high serum
protein binding. The $-CH_2$ CH NH_2 COOH substituted molecule is very interesting
because, although its partition coefficient is very low (0.02), the BUI is quite
high (24.3%) suggesting a carrier mediated transport (50).

In addition to these types of compounds, other neutral chelates as PIPSE
and MOSE can diffuse through BBB into the cells where the pH is lower (7.0-7.1):
because of the pH shift they pick up an H ion, become charged and are no
longer lipid soluble; therefore, they cannot diffuse out of the cells (51).
According to this general principle it should be possible to obtain a Tc-compound
starting from a Tc-molecule as bis (2 mercaptoethyl) amine (52).

REFERENCES

1. Atkins HL et al.In: Radiopharmaceuticals II, The Society of Nuclear Medici
   Sorenson JA (ed), New York, 1979, p. 183.

2. Front D, J. Neurol. Neurosurg. Psychiat. 41:18, 1978.

3. Washburn LC et al. J. nucl. Med. 22:75, 1981 (abstract).

4. Nahmias C et al. J. nucl. Med. 16:676, 1975.

5. Glenn HJ et al. In: Radiopharmaceuticals II, The Society of Nuclear Medici
   Sorensen JA (ed), New York, 1979, p. 285.

6. Sugitani Y et al. J. nucl. Med. 14:912, 1973.

7. Schwartz ML, Tator CH, J. nucl. Med. 13:321, 1972.

8. Tator CH, In: Radiopharmaceuticals, The Society of Nuclear Medicine,
   Subramanian G, Rhodes BA, Cooper JF, Sodd VJ (eds), New York, 1975, p. 474

9. Jenkinson IS et al, Int. J. Nucl. Med. Biol. 2:175, 1975.

10. Bernes I et al. Strahlentherapie 74:107, 1975, (Sonderb.).

11. Waxman AD et al. J. nucl. Med. 17:345, 1976.

12. Mamo L et al. Nouv. Press Méd. 11:795, 1975.

13. Fisher KC et al. J. nucl. Med. 16:705, 1975.

14. Brambilla GL et al. In: Proc. 2nd Nat. Meet. of SIRMN, Rome, 1977, p. 115.

15. Brambilla G et al. Acta Neurochir. 36:165, 1977 (abstract).

16. Ectors M et al. J. nucl. Med. 16:526, 1975 (abstract).

17. Sager WD et al, J. nucl. Med. 16:257, 1977.

18. Rollo FD et al. Radiology 123:379, 1977.

19. Tanasescu DE et al. Radiology 130:421, 1979.

20. Tanasescu DE et al. J. nucl. Med. 19:673, 1978 (abstract).

21. Tanasescu DE et al. J. nucl. Med. 18:630, 1977 (abstract).

22. Leveille J et al. J. nucl. Med. 18:957, 1977.

23. Aprile C, Favino A, In: Progress in Radiopharmacology, Vol. II, Cox PH (ec
    Elsevier/North-Holland Biomedical Press, Amsterdam, 1981, p.327.

24. Boyd RE et al. Brit. J. Radiol. 46:604, 1973.

25. Favino A, Aprile C, In: Progress in Radiopharmacology, Vol. I, Cox PH (ed)
    Elsevier/North-Holland Biomedical Press, Amsterdam, 1979, p. 75.

26. Akerman M et al. J. nucl. Med. 18:630, 1977 (abstract).

27. Ell PJ et al. Proc. 13th Ann. Meet. Soc. Nucl. Med. Copenhagen, 1975.

28. Kim EE et al. J. nucl. Med. 21:838, 1980.

29. Ryo UY et al. J. nucl. Med. 16:127, 1975.

30. Mori T et al. J. nucl. Med. 16:414, 1975.

31. Odori T, Jap. J. Nucl. Med. 16:721, 1979.

32. Hurley PJ, J. nucl. Med. 13:156, 1972.

33. Waxman AD et al, J. nucl. Med. 15:524, 1974 (abstract).

34. Hill TC et al. J. nucl. Med. 18:877, 1977.

35. Hays MT, Green FA, J. nucl. Med. 14:149, 1973.

36. Dewanjee MK, In: Radiopharmaceuticals II, The Society of Nuclear Medicine, Sorenson JA (ed), New York, 1979, p. 435.

37. Dewanjee MK, In: Principles of Radiopharmacology, Vol. III, Colombetti LG (ed), CRC Press, Boca Raton, USA, 1979, p. 61.

38. Cox PH, Van der Pompe WB, In: Progress in Radiopharmacology, Vol. I, Cox PH (ed), Elsevier/North-Holland Biomedical Press, Amsterdam, 1979, p. 45.

39. Aprile C et al. Proc. 19th Ann. Meet. Soc. Nucl. Med. Bern, 1981, p. 251, (abstract).

40. Pompe Van der WB, In: Progress in Radiopharmacology, Vol. I, Cox PH (ed), Elsevier/North-Holland Biomedical Press, Amsterdam, 1979, p. 31.

41. Hunt FC, Personal Communication, 1980.

42. Anghileri LJ, In: Principles of Radiopharmacology, Vol. III, Colombetti LG (ed), CRC Press, Boca Raton, USA, 1979, p. 243.

43. Kuhl DE et al. Circulat. Res. 36:610, 1975.

44. Grubb RL et al. Ann. Neurol. 4:322, 1978.

45. Kuhl DE et al. J. Neurosurg. 52:309, 1980.

46. Phelps ME et al. J. nucl. Med. 20:328, 1979.

47. Verhas M et al, J. nucl. Med. 17:170, 1976.

48. Etani H et al. J. nucl. Med. 22:856, 1981.

49. Oldendorf WH, Ann. Neurol. 10:207, 1981.

50. Loberg MD et al. In: Radiopharmaceuticals II, The Society of Nuclear Medicine, Sorenson JA (ed), New York, 1979, p. 449.

51. Kung HF, Blau M, J. nucl. Med. 21:147, 1980.

52. Burns HD et al, J. nucl. Med. 20:654, 1979 (abstract).

MEASUREMENT OF REGIONAL CEREBRAL FUNCTION FOR NEUROLOGICAL RESEARCH USING POSITRON EMISSION TOMOGRAPHY AND SHORTlIVED CYCLOTRON PRODUCED ISOTOPES

C.G. RHODES

INTRODUCTION

Advances in the understanding of brain pathophysiology and the treatment of cerebral disorders are, in many respects, restricted by the development of associated technologies. This is illustrated by the paucity of reliable measurements of regional cerebral function which, until recently, have been limited to measurements of blood flow and of the general integrity of the blood brain barrier - using indicator dilution techniques and radioactive tracers. The restricted development of these techniques has been due to the virtual lack of spatial resolution of the various imaging devices in the depth plane and the limited choice of radio-actively labelled tracers.

However, with the development of positron emission totmography, it is now possible to accurately measure the regional distribution of the concentration of positron emitting isotopes with a spatial resolution (in three dimensions) of between 10 and 16mm (full width at half maximum). In addition, many of the cyclotron produced isotopes can be incorporated into biologically relevant compounds, which range from the relatively simple molecules $^{15}O_2$ and $H_2^{15}O$ to the more complex glucose analogues (^{18}F-deoxyglucose and ^{11}C-methylglucose), amino acids)^{11}C-leucine and ^{11}C-methionine) and brain receptor labels (^{11}C-etorphine and ^{11}C-pimozide). Great importance is also attached to the extremely short half life of some of these isotopes which allows them to be used to measure dynamic functions (such as blood flow) under steady state conditions using constant infusion or inhalation techniques (1,2). Thus it is possible to measure a variety of regional functional parameters in the brain of man non - invasively and atraumatically in the clinical environment (3). This highlights the principal investigative power of the field, namely to provide analytical means for piecing together the complex patho-physiological picture.

In this paper, the methodologies required for the measurement of blood flow (using $C^{15}O_2$), oxygen and glucose metabolism (using $^{15}O_2$ and ^{18}F-labelled fluorodeoxyglucose) and blood volume (using ^{11}CO) are described, and the clini- cal and scientific relevance of such measurements illustrated by considering results taken from studies of two important focal brain diseases - cerebral glioma and stroke.

METHODOLOGIES

Measurement of blood flow and oxygen consumption

Measurements of regional cerebral blood flow (rCBF), oxygen extraction (rOER) and the rate of oxygen metabolism (rCMRO$_2$) are obtained using the steady state oxygen-15 inhalation technique first described by Jones et al (1). This technique requires the constant inhalation of two gases labelled with oxygen- carbon dioxide ($C^{15}O_2$) and molecular oxygen itself ($^{15}O_2$). The constant inhala- tion of $C^{15}O_2$ results in the labelling of $H_2{}^{15}O$ in the lung capillaries (4) and an eventual steady state concentration of activity in the systemic arterial blood. Since the half-life of oxygen-15 only 2.05 min, the tissue concentration of this tracer does not reach the equilibrium level of the arterial blood because of the finite transit time of the tracer through the extravascular tissue water pool. Equating the input of tracer to this pool, via the arterial blood, to the loss of tracer by virtue of venous outflow and radioactive decay "en route" through the tissue mass, results in the equation

$$C_{t_1} = C_{a_1} \frac{F/V}{F/V + \lambda}$$

where C_{t_1} and C_{a_1} are the tissue and arterial blood concentrations of $H_2{}^{15}O$ respectively, F/V is the blood flow per unit volume of tissue (rCBF) and λ is the radioactive decay constant for oxygen-15 (0.337 min^{-1}).

During the inhalation of $^{15}O_2$ the nwe tissue concentration of $H_2{}^{15}O$ (C_{t_2} results mainly from the "water of metabolism" which is the end-product of the metabolism of the $^{15}O_2$ extracted from the arterial blood (C_{a_2}). Thus a second equation can be constructed which incorporates the oxygen extraction ratio (OER), thus

$$C_{t_2} - C_{a_2} \frac{F/V \ OER}{F/V + \lambda}$$

Provided C_{t_1}, C_{t_2}, C_{a_2} can be measured in the same units the two equations can be solved to give rCBF (F/V) and rOER. Blood sampling allows both the measurement of C_{a_1} and C_{a_2}, and O_c, the arterial blood oxygen content, which then allows the rate of oxygen metabolism to be calculated using the equation

$$rCMRO_2 = rCBF \cdot rOER \cdot O_c$$

In practice, modifications have to be made to the second equation to account for the recirculating water of metabolism from other organs in the body and for the molecular oxygen-15 bound to the red blood cells in the brain tissue. (These aspects are incorporated in the operational equations of the oxygen-15 inhalation technique but have been omitted here for brevity).

Measurements of the regional tissue isotope concentration are made using a positron tomograph (E.G. and G. ORTEC ECAT II). Concidence detection of the paired monoenergetic 511 KeV gamma rays, which result from the positron annihilation (figue 1), allows a tomographic reconstruction of the original isotope distribution to be made with a spatial resolution of 16mm. If a correction for tissue attenuation of the emitted photons is incorporated into the reconstruction algorithm (using information obtained from a transmission scan recorded during the exposure of an external positron emitting ring source), the resulting tomograph provides a quantitative distribution of the isotope concentration. This instrument has been shown to have a linear response to isotope concentration with no zero offset. The two scans recorded during the inhalation of $C^{15}O_2$ and $^{15}O_2$ are converted from values of $H_2^{15}O$ concentration (C_{t1} and C_{t2}) to values of rCBF, rOER and $rCMRO_2$ using the equations described by Frackowiak et al (5). The sentivity of this method for following changes in rCBF and $rCMRO_2$ has been studied experimentally by Rhodes et al (6) and Baron et al (7). In addition, the uncertainties introduced by compounding the various statistical errors have been reported by Lammertsma et al (8) who have also expanded on the original treatise of Frackowiak et al (9).

Measurement of Glucose Metabolism

Measurements of glucose metabolism (rCMRglu) are made using a modified version of the general deoxyglucose technique of Sokoloff et al (10) which was later adapted by Phelps et al (11) for use with positron emission tomography using fluorine-18 labelled 2-fluoro-2-deoxy-D-glucose (FDG). FDG is a glucose

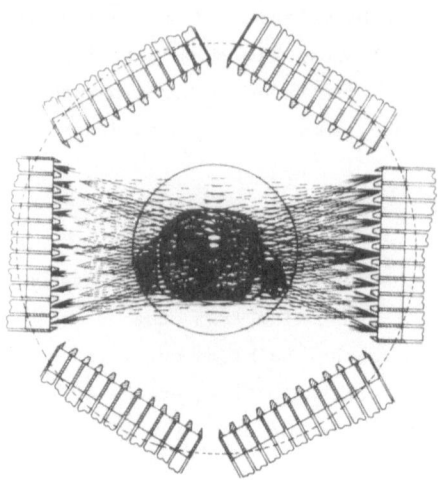

Fig. 1. Hexagonal configuration of the 66 NaI detectors of the E.G. and G. ORT
ECAT II. Each detector is in electronic coincidence with the eleven detectors
the opposing bank, thus providing adequate sparial sampling over the field of
view (inner circle).

analogue which competes with glucose for transport across the blood brain barr
and phosphorylation by the intracellular enzyme hexokinase, but is not metabolised further because of its altered chemical structure. The resulting fluoro-
deoxyglucose-6-phosphate (FDG-6-P) is then effectivly trapped in the tissue
since its rate of hydrolysis (dephosphorylation) is very low. Although the ear
isotope concentration in the brain tissue, following an intravenous injection,
is mainly unphosphorylated FDG, the turnover rate of this species is measured
minutes and with the progressive elimination of FDG from the plasma pool, the
tissue activit at times greater than 50-60 minutes is predominantly intracellu
FDG-6-P. Thus the equation of Sokloff and Phelps can be approximated by the
equation.

$$rCMRglu = C_i^*(T) C_p / LC \int_o^T C_p^*(t) dt$$

where $C_i^*(T)$ is the tissue concentration of radiotracer at a time T after the
intravenous injection of FDG, $C_p^*(t)$ is the arterial blood plasma concentration
of FDG at time t, C_p^* is the steady stae plasma glucose concentration of the
arterial blood and LC, the lumped constant, relates the handling of FDG and
glucose by the brain tissue.

Measurements of regional blood volume (rCBV) are made using carbon-11 labelled carbon monoxide (^{11}CO) (12). This tracer is administered as a bolus inhalation which labels the red cells of the lung capillaries. Emission scans are recorded following a five minute equilibration period to allow the mixing of these red cells with the systemic blood volume. The regional blood volume measurement not only provides useful information on the degree of regional vascularisation of the cerebral tissue but is necessary for the blood volume correction of the calculated rOER values (9).

Relationship between rCBF, rCMRO$_2$ and rCMRglu

Whilst the measurement of what can be termed "primary" function, namely rCBF, rCMRO$_2$ and rCMRglu, undoubtedly provides useful information about the status of brain tissue, it is the relationship between these parameters which gives a specific insight into the physiological disturbances of pathology. These relationships are derived from the comparison between the rates of oxygen and glucose metabolism and their supply, to provide regional extraction ratios for oxygen and glucose (rOER and rGER respectively), and from the comparison between the rates of oxygen and glucose metabolism themselves, to provide regional values of the metabolic ratio (rMR = rCMRO$_2$/rCMRglu).

In normal brain tissue the rOER values are well defined (varying between 0.35 and 0.45) with no detectable differences between grey and white matter (figure 2). Thus, under normal conditions, the tissues have a moderate reserve of oxygen supply. However, two abnormal states are now well recognised - 1. luxury perfusion, where there is a disproportionately high blood flow to meet the metabolic demand, as manifest by low values of rOER, and 2. critical perfusion, where there is a disproportionately low blood flow to meet the metabolic demand. This second state, which is characterised by substantially increased values of rOER, includes both ischaemia - where there is insufficient blood supply to meet the metabolic need of the tissue, and diminished perfusion reserve - where the tissue's metabolic demand has not yet been compromised by the reduced blood flow but is dangerously close. It is important to realise that luxury perfusion may be associated with low rCBF if rCMRO$_2$ is reduced to a disproportionately greater extent - a common pattern in established cerebral infarction. Therefore, defining a low rCBF alone cannot differentiate between ischaemia or infarction, two very different pathophysiological states.

The metabolic ratio (rCMRO$_2$/rCMRglu) is also thought to be relatively constant in normal cerebral tissue with values ranging from 0.6 to 0.7 (mg-glucose)$^{-1}$

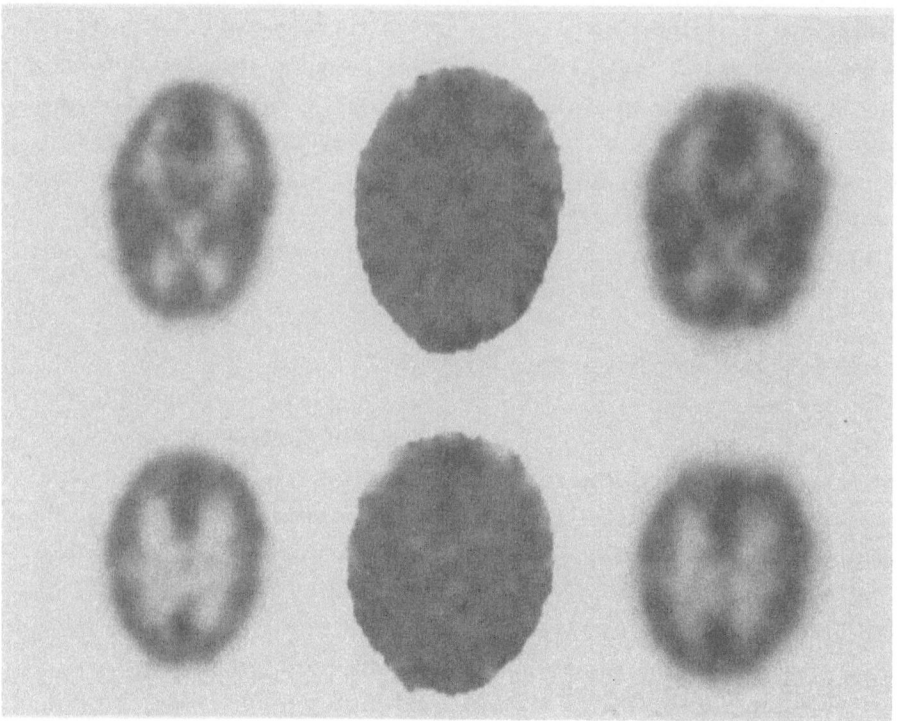

Fig. 2. Functional tomographic images of rCBF (left), rOER (centre) and rCMRO (right) measured at standard levels through the brain of a normal subject. Lower: - orbitomeatal (OM) line + 4 cm plane, Upper: - OM + 6 cm plane. The subjects left is to the left of the image, anterior is to the top. Each functional image is displayed such that its highest value is represented by t maximum on the grey scale.

(derived from values of global $CMRO_2$ and CMRqlu taken from the literature). A increase in this parameter is indicative of the aerobic metabolism of nutrien in addition to glucose, whilst a decrease in its value indicates anaerobic glycolysis.

Cerebral function in glioma and stroke

To illustrate the sizeable impact of these techniques in neurological research, fuctional measurements made on patients with cerebral glioma and stroke are considered.

Functional images are shown for representive studies from the two patien groups in Figure 3. Numerical analysis of the tomographic data from each stud was performed to obtain mean values of the various functional parameters for discrete brain regions representative of tumour and contralateral grey for the group 1 (glioma) patients, and infarcted tissue and contralateral cortex for the group 2 (stroke) patients.

Blood flow in the region of the glioma was found to be substantial - comparable to that in the contralateral grey - but $rCMRO_2$ was depressed. This resulted in low values of rOER. In contrast, however, tumour rCMRglu was maintained at levels that related to the rCBF and resulted in normal rGER values for both glioma and the contralateral grey tissue. No difference was observed between the mean rCBV values for the two regions of the group 1 patients.

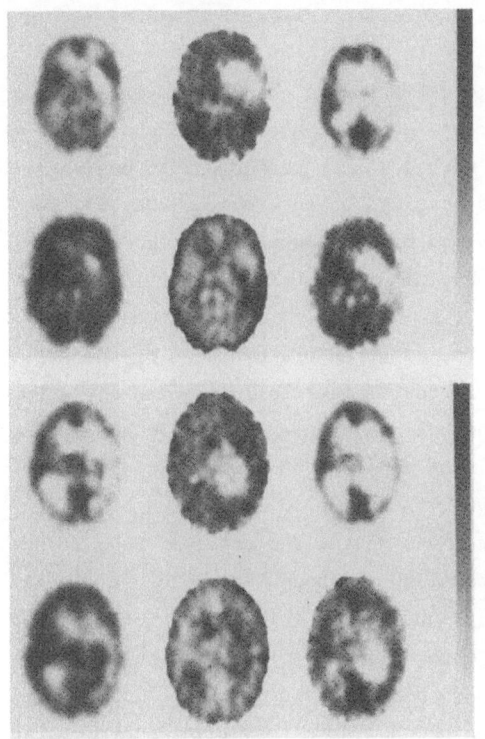

Fig. 3. Functional tomographic images obtained from (a) a patient with a recurrent grade 4 astrocytoma (right hemisphere) and (b) a stroke patient 4 days following the onset of symptoms. In each set of images the functional parameters displayed are: Upper (leftlright) rCBF, rOER and $rCMRO_2$, Lower (left-right) rCMRglu, rGER and rMR (= $rCMRO_2/rCMRglu$). The abnormalities seen in these analogue displays are typical of those for the patient groups as a whole and are described in the text. However, note the mismatching between rCBF and $rCMRO_2$ and rCMRglu, as defined by low values of rOER and rGER respectively.

The disparity between the tumour $rCMRO_2$ and rCMRglu, as reflected by the low rMR, indicated that cells in the region of the glioma were metabolising glucose anaerobically since only half the normal amount of oxygen was being consumed per mg of glucose (compared to a normal rMR in the contralateral grey matter). This could be important from the therapeutic point of view since it strongly suggests a lowering of local tissue pH. The finding of low rOER in cerebral gliomas has interesting implications since it means that the end capillary blood has an elevated oxygen content (relative to normal tissue whic have a higher rOER) and that, at the macroscopic level at least, the tissue is not hypoxic and does not, therefore, have the radiotherapeutic disadvantage of being radioinsensitive.

The results of the studies on stroke patients are characterised by extrem low values of $rCMRO_2$ in the infarcted areas. However, the rCBF, though low, wa not coupled to $rCMRO_2$ and resulted in a marked luxury perfusion. In contrast, rCMRglu was less depressed than rCBF and resulted in an elevated rGER in the infarcted area compared to the normal values of the contralateral cortex. In these group 2 studies there was a small but significant fall (30%) in the rCBV of the infarcted tissue.

The general finding of low rOER in the affected brain tissue of the strok patients shows quite clearly that, in a matter of days following the catastrop fall in regional cerebral blood flow, the balance between metabolic supply and demand is heavily weighted in favour of rCBF and that the tissue is no longer ischaemic. Because of the disparity between the rates of oxygen and glucose metabolism, the rMR of the infarcted area was severely depressed, suggesting high proportion of anaerobic glucose metabolism (although some glucose may hav been used in synthetic pathways for the production of amino acids, etc.). Whil some degree of anaerobic metabolism may expected in the ischaemic period follc ing the stroke, it is difficult to envisage how this could persist for days, especially in view of the very low oxygen demand. An alternative interpretatic of these results is that the substantial rate of glucose metabolism orginates not from the "indigenous" brain tissue, but from invading macrophages or neu-trophils which are part of the healing process and are known to metabolise glucose anaerobically for a major part of their energy requirements (13). On t other hand, it may be that the reliance on the use of a glucose analogue and such a relatively simple model for the measurement of rCMRglu, is, in such extreme conditions, inappropriate. The quantitative analysis of this work is currently being prepared for publication.

Conclusion

Whilst the various aspects of neurological research covered in this presentation are by no means fully comprehensive, they do give a general insight into the methodologies involved and their role in the gathering of clinical scientific information. The use of positron emission tomography provides the ability to quantitate the regional isotope concentration, with a high degree of spatial accuracy, thus allowing the cyclotron produced isotopes to be used in new and exciting ways to measure a wide variety of physiological functtios. Therefore, it is quite realistic to consider the use of these techniques as a means for rationalising and testing the efficiency of therapeutic regimes, with the aim of broadening the general understanding of the impact of proposed treatment regimes on pathological processes in common neurological disorders.

Acknowledgements

The studies described in this presentation form part of the neurological research programme at the MRC Cyclotron Unit and directly involved the active collaboration of Drs. R.J.S. Wise, J.M. Gibbs, J. Hatazawa, R.S.J. Frackowiak and T. Jones. We would like to thank Mr. D.D. Vonberg, the Director, and the many other members of the Unit for their invaluable support, especially Dr. A.J. Palmer and Mr. P.D. Buckingham for the preparation of radiolabelled materials.

REFERENCES

1. Jones T, Chester DA, Ter-Pogossian MM. (1976): The continuous inhalation of oxygen-15 for assessing regional oxygen extraction in the brain of man. Br. J. Radiol. 49:339-343.

2. Huang SC, Phelps ME, Hoffman EJ, Kuhl DE. (1979): A theoretical study of quantitative flow measurements with constant infusion of short-lived isotope Phys. Med. Biol. 24:1151-1161.

3. Phelps ME, Mazziotta JC, Huang SC. (1982): Study of cerebral function with positron computed tomography - Review. J. Cereb. Blood Flow Metab. 2: 113-162.

4. West JB, Dollery CT. (1962): Uptake of oxygen-15 labelled CO_2 compared with carbon-11 labelled CO_2 in the lung. J. Appl. Physiol. 17:9-13.

5. Frackowiak RSJ, Lenzi GL, Jones T, Heather JD. (1980): Quantitative measurement of regional cerebral blood flow and oxygen metabolism in man using ^{15}O and positron emission tomography: Theory, procedure and normal values. J. Comput Assist. Tomogr. 4:727-736.

6. Rhodes CG, Lenzi GL, Frackowiak RSJ, Jones T, Pozzili C. (1981): Measurement of CBF and $CMRO_2$ using the continuous inhalation of $C^{15}O_2$ and $^{15}O_2$:Experimental validation using CO_2 reactivity in the anaesthetised dog. J. Neurol. Sci. 50 381-389.

7. Baron JC, Steinling M, Tanaka T, Cavalheiro E, Soussaline F, Collard P. (1981): Quantitative measurement of CBF, oxygen extraction fraction (OEF) and $CMRO_2$ with ^{15}O continuous inhalation techniques and positron emission tomography (PET): Experimental evidence and normal values in man. J.Cereb. Blood Flow Metabol., 1(Suppl.1):55-56.

8. Lammertsma AA, Heather JD, Jones T, Frackowiak RSJ, Lenzi GL. (1982): A statistical study of the steady state technique for measuring regional cerebral blood flow and oxygen utilisation using ^{15}O. J. Comput. Assist. Tomogr. 6(3):566-573.

9. Lammertsma AA, Jones T, Frackowiak RSJ, Lenzi GL. (1981): A theoretical study of the steady state model for measuring regional cerebral blood flow and oxygen utilisation using oxygen-15. J. Comput Assist Tomogr. 5:544-550.

10. Sokoloff L, Reivich M, Kennedy C, Des Rosiers MH, Patlak CS, Pettigrew KD, Sakurada KD, Sakurada O.(1977): The (^{14}C)-dexyglucose method for the measurement of local cerebral glucose utilisation: Theory, procedure and normal values in the conscious and anesthetised rat. J. Neurochem. 28:897-916.

11. Phelps ME, Huang SC, Hoffman EJ, Kuhl DE. (1979): Tomographic measurement of local cerebral glucose metabolic rate in humans with (F-18) 2-fluoro-2-deoxy D-glucose: Validation of method. Ann. Neurol. 6:371-388.

12. Phelps ME, Huang SC, Hoffman EJ, Kuhl DE. (1979): Tomographic measurement of cerebral blood volume C-11 labelled carboxyhemoglobin. J. Nucl. Med.20:328-3

13. Cline MJ. (1975): The White Cell. Harvard University Press, pp.39-70, 479-48

3-(^{11}C)-METHYL-D-GLUCOSE, AN AGENT FOR THE ASSESSMENT OF REGIONAL GLUCOSE TRANSPORT ACROSS THE BLOOD-BRAIN BARRIER

G. KLOSTER, G. STÖCKLIN, K. VYSKA, C. FREUNDLIEB, A. HÖCK,
L.E. FEINENDEGEN, H. TRAUPE, W.D. HEISS

INTRODUCTION

The normal brain meets its energy needs solely by oxidative metabolism of D-glucose. Thus, labelled derivatives of D-glucose may be expected to be useful tracers for glucose utilization. Since D-glucose cannot freely enter the brain, but instead uses a carrier-mediated diffusion system (the hexose carrier), strict stereochemical requirements have to be met by D-glucose tracer analogues. The electronegative substituents must be in an all-cis as well as an all-equatorial configuration. Thus, all the analogues investigated so far, have that particular arrangement. Raichle et al. (1,2) studied the distribution of photo-synthetically prepared ^{11}C-D-glucose in monkeys. However, the multiple pathways of glucose metabolism present made it very difficult to interpret the data accumulated during the in vivo measurements. Ido et al. (3) synthetized the D-glucose analogue ^{18}F-2-fluoro-2-deoxy-D-glucose (FDG) and the biodistribution was studied in mice by Gallagher et al. (4). FDG was successfully applied to the measurement of regional glucose metabolic rates in man by Reivich et al. (5) and Phelps et al. (6). FDG is transported into the brain via the hexose carrier; once inside the cell it is phosphorylated by hexokinase to yield FDG-6-phosphate which cannot be further utilized for glucolysis. FDG is thus trapped inside the cell. This is an in vivo application of the well-known autoradiographic ^{14}C-2-deoxy-D-glucose method of Sokoloff et al. (7). Using any of these methods (3-7), an integral value of regional cerebral glucose utilization is obtained for the time period between administration of the radiopharmaceutical and recording of the data using a positron emission tomograph (PET). Other possible compounds using the same approach are ^{18}F-3-fluoro-3-deoxy-D-glucose (8,9) and ^{11}C-2-deoxy-D-glucose (10).

It was felt that a tracer was needed which makes differential measurements of changes in regional cerebral glucose utilization possible, i.e., a tracer is desirable that is not metabolically trapped inside the cell. Such a tracer is ^{11}C-3-Methyl-D-glucose (MG) (11-15). MG is transported from blood into brain by

the same carrier as D-glucose and the K_M's for both compounds are nearly iden
tical (13,14). MG is not metabolized at all (15), but is excreted unchanged v
the kidneys. We report here that these useful characteristics of MG allow
simultaneous dynamic in vivo measurements of regional cerebral glucose transp
rate and local perfusion using PET (16,17).

Radiopharmaceutical

MG was synthetized from the commercially available 1,2:5,6-diisopropylic
D-glucose via the potassium salt by methylation using [11]CH_3I (18). Hydrolysis
the ketal groups yields MG (fig. 1). After analysis by high pressure liquid
chromatography, purification and dissolution in saline, MG is ready for injec
tion. The overall yield after sterile filtration was 35 % with a mean prepara
tion time of 34 min (11,12). Recently, this synthesis was adapted to a remote
control apparatus in order to reduce the radiation dose to the chemist (19).
Thus, batches of 3-8 mCi MG can be produced reproducibly.

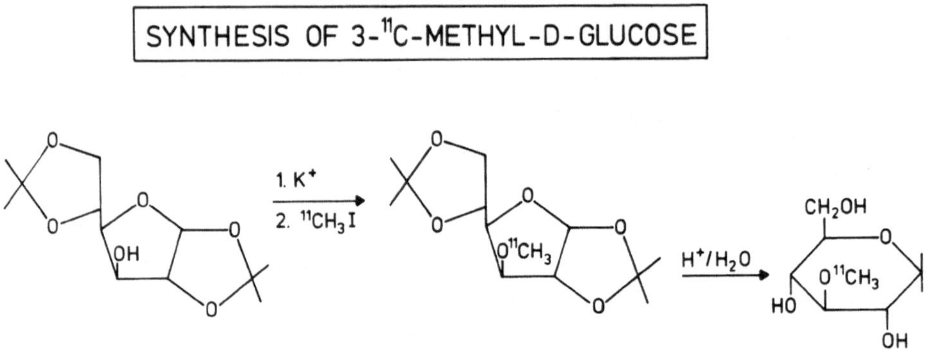

SYNTHESIS OF 3-^{11}C-METHYL-D-GLUCOSE

Fig. 1.

Biodistribution in animals

After i.v. injection of 1-10 µCi MG into female NMRI albino mice, all well perfused organs such as lung, heart, kidney and brain rapidly accumulate MG. The accumulation in the brain is significant for the time interval between administration and 15 min after administration. At 15 min, the concentration of radioactivity in brain is 175% mean body concentration (%MBC) $\hat{=}$ 6.2% dose/g organ. The brain-to blood-ratio rises to about 0.7 during the same time inter- val. This compares favourably with data obtained with ^{3}H-MG by Wassenaar et al. (20). It is less than in the case of FDG (4), where about 18% dose/g brain was found. However since we are investigating a tracer which can be transported back and forth through the blood-brain-barrier (13) this difference is not surprising.

These data were confirmed in in vivo experiments in rabbits using a γ- camera (21). Again, the main accumulation was in heart, liver, kidney and the brain, although the brain is less clearly visualized than the other organs mentioned. MG is rapidly concentrated in the kidneys and excreted via the urine (11,12,15,20). Hence, in addition to the short physical half-life of ^{11}C, the biological half-time is also short, thus reducing the radiation dose to the patient.

Investigations in patients

After i.v. injection of 2-6 mCi MG into an antecubital vein, the transaxial activity in the head of the patient was registered with the ECAT II Scanner at 2 min intervals for 40 min. The images were taken in one slice selected according to the pathological areas in the X-ray CT scan (17,22,23). MG was found to be effectively accumulated in normal brain cortex, significantly lower accumulation was observed in white matter (fig. 2).

Among 20 patients with stroke, with a total of 26 ischemic areas, the size of the MG accumulation defects closely resembled those detected as hypodense areas in CT-scans in 10 areas. In 16 areas the ischemic defects appeared to be larger than in CT (fig. 3). These results indicate that in patients suffering from ischemic stroke larger brain areas had been affected by stroke than was suggested by CT. One of the possible reasons for the deactivation of morphologi- cally intact cerebral cortex may be the interruption of coritical fiber tracts/24). This conclusion seems to be supported by the observation made in a patient who had left homonymous hemianopia which was caused by infarction in the right middle cerebral artery (fig. 4). No ischemia was apparent in the territory of

202

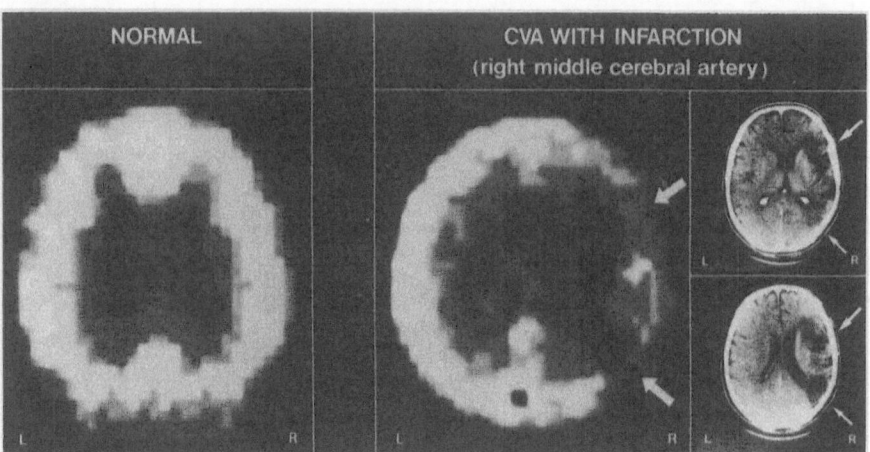

NORMAL

CVA WITH INFARCTION
(right middle cerebral artery)

L R

Figures 2 and 3

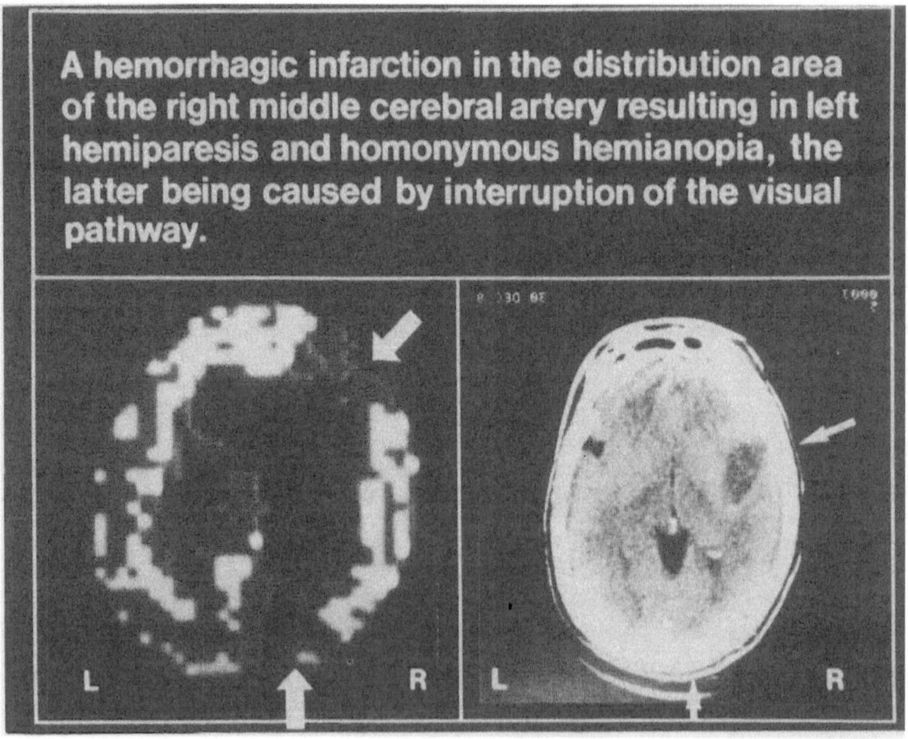

A hemorrhagic infarction in the distribution area
of the right middle cerebral artery resulting in left
hemiparesis and homonymous hemianopia, the
latter being caused by interruption of the visual
pathway.

L R L R

Figure 4

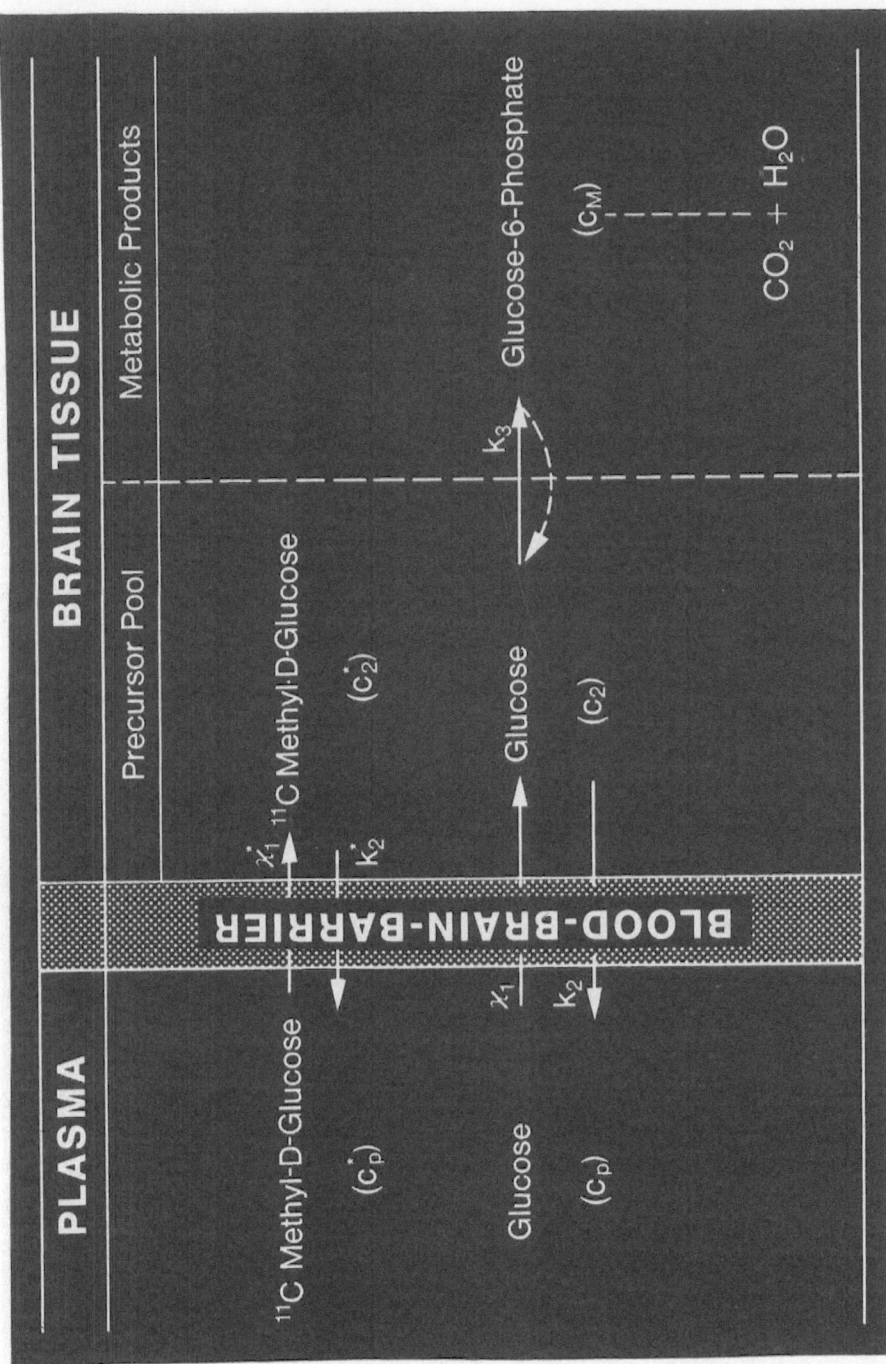

Figure 5

of the posterior cerebral artery which supplies the visual cortex. In the MG
study of this patient two accumulation defects were observed. One was frontal
and corresponded to the hypodense area observed in CT. The second, in the ips
lateral primary and associative visual cortex, had no CT correlate. This defe
demonstrated the response of the visual cortex to the destruction of visual
pathways.

Simultaneous quantification of regional perfusion and local glucose
transport rate

Following i.v. application, MG competes with plasma glucose for transpor
from plasma into a common primary precursor pool in brain tissue via the hexo
carrier of the blood brain barrier (13,14) (fig. 5). Inside the cell most of
glucose is phosphorylated and further metabolized, while a small portion of
glucose together with the non-metabolizable MG (15) is transported back into
circulation by the same carrier. Since MG is not metabolized the rate of its
accumulation in brain tissue dc_2*/dt is equal to the difference between MG
influx and MG efflux.

$$\frac{dc_2^*}{dt} = \phi_i^* - \phi_e^* \tag{A}$$

MG influx

ϕ_i^* is directly proportional to the amount of available MG supplied to tl
tissue per unit time (q_A^*) (25,26,27), i.e.

$$\phi_i^* = k_1^* \, q_A^* \tag{B}$$

where $\bar{k}_1^*$ is the proportionality constant reflecting the catalytic activity o
the carrier system for influx of MG.

MG does not readily enter erythrocytes (28). Thus, all MG injected stays
plasma and can thus be utilized for transmembrane transport. Consequently, q_A
is given by the product between blood MG concentration c_B^* and the local perfu
sion rate f_i. Thus,

$$\phi_i^* = k_1^* \, f_i \, c_B^* \tag{C}$$

Because the perfused brain is a semi-open system with no instantaneous mixing and not a closed system such as tissue culture, not only the catalytic activity of the carrier for MG influx but also the local perfusion rate determines the observed rate constant for MG influx (K_1^*). Thus

$$K_1^* = k_1^* \, f_i \qquad (D)$$

and

$$\phi_i^* = K_1^* \, c_B^* \qquad (E)$$

MG efflux

ϕ_e^* is directly proportional to the MG concentration in brain tissue c_2^* (7)

$$\phi_e^* = k_2^* \, c_2^* \qquad (F)$$

where k_2^* reflects the catalytic activity of the carrier for MG efflux.

MG tissue concentration

By substituting (F) and (E) into (A), one obtains

$$\frac{dc_2^*}{dt} = K_1^* \, c_B^* - k_2^* \, c_2^* \qquad (G)$$

On integration, one obtains

$$c_2^*(t) = K_1^* \, (\int c_B^*(\tau) \, e^{k_2^* \tau} \, d\tau + \eta) \, e^{-k_2^* t} \qquad (H)$$

where η is the integration constant.

Equation (H) relates c_B^*, K_1^* and k_2^+ to c_2^*. Since c_2^* and c_B^* can be directly obtained from time-activity-curves (fig.6) this equation permits the determination of K_1^* and k_2^* in any selected brain area (for details see 17,29).

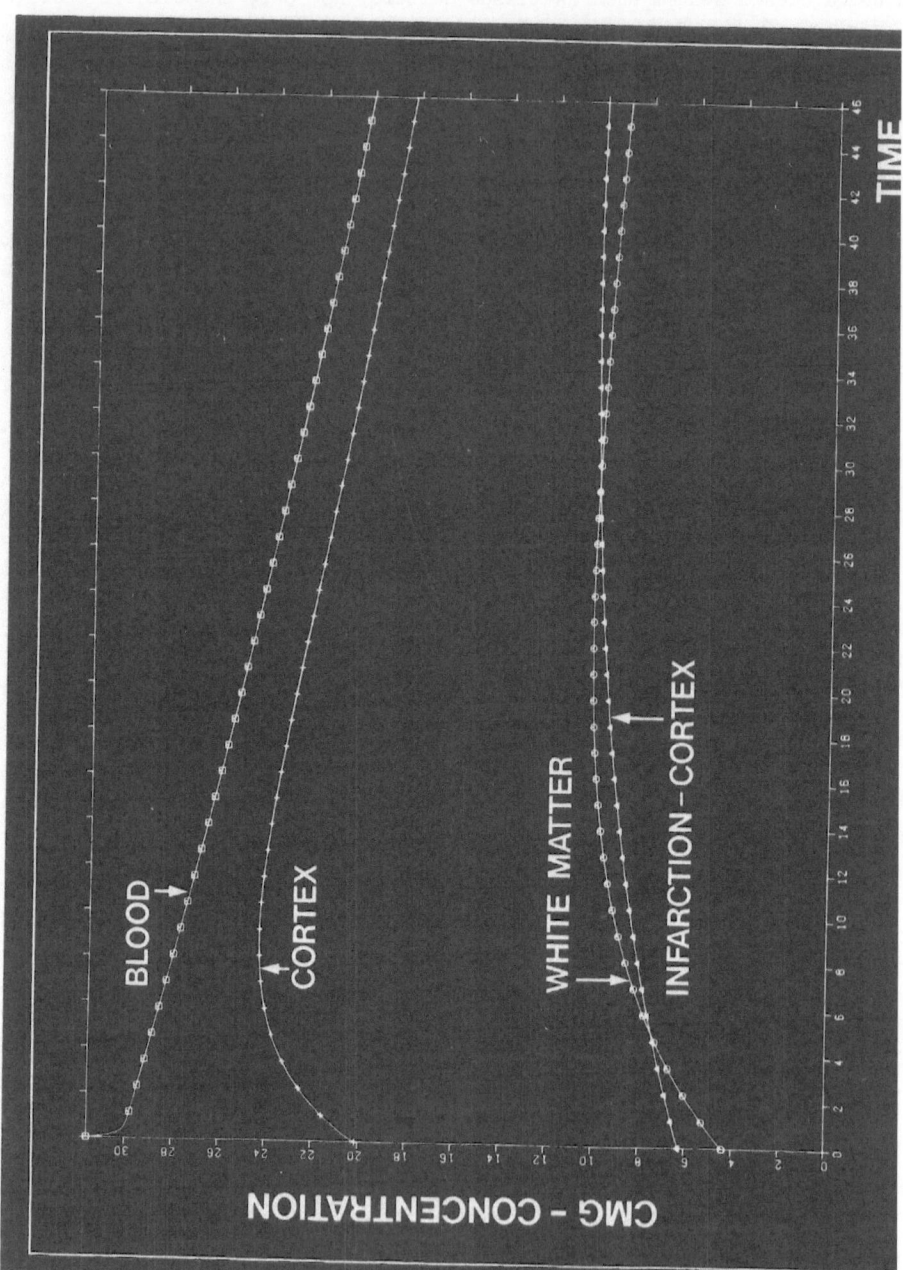

Local perfusion rate

On dividing equation (D) by k_2^*, one obtains

$$\frac{K_1^*}{k_2^*} = f_i \, \frac{k_1^*}{k_2^*} \qquad (I)$$

Hence, the ratio K_1^*/k_2^* is equal to the product of the local perfusion rate f_i and the ratio of the constants k_1^* and k_2^*. If we make the simplifying assumption $k_1^* = k_2^*$, one obtains

$$f_i = \frac{K_1^*}{k_2^*} \qquad (K)$$

This means that, using this assumption, the ratio K_1^*/k_2^* is a quantitative expression of local perfusion rate. It was shown (17,29) that the local perfusion rate f_i closely agrees with data obtained by other techniques (5,30,31).

Local glucose transport rate

In a similar manner to the method used for MG the rate of glucose influx can be derived as (17,29):

$$\phi_i = K_1 (1 - H_t) \, c_p, \qquad (L)$$

c_p being the plasma glucose concentration, H_t the blood hematocrit and K_1 the observed rate constant for glucose influx. H_t and c_p can be determined by blood analysis, whereas k_1 must be obtained from MG time-activity-curves. Data obtained in rats by Pardridge and Oldendorf (13) led to the result (17,29)

$$K_1 = 1.11 \, K_1^* \qquad (M)$$

Thus, the local glucose transport rate is

$$\phi_i = 1.11 \, K_1^* (1 - h_t) \, c_p \qquad (N)$$

Quantitative results in patients

Typical time-activity-curves detected over the superior longitudinal sinus and over different regions of the brain are demonstrated in fig. 6. The activity registered over the superior longitudinal sinus was considered to represent the concentration of MG in blood and was used as the input function.

The blood-curve usually showed two exponential components. The initial rapid decrease of activity probably reflects mixing of the indicator in the blood-pool; this was followed by a slow elimination phase, indicating good retention of the non-metabolizable tracer in blood.

Time-activity-curves registered over different brain regions shows a rapid accumulation and a slow elimination phase. Accumulation half-times in normal brain ranged from 1.8 - 3.2 min for cortex and 5-7 min for white matter. They were significantly prolonged for ischemic areas, exceeding 10 min in cortex and 16 min in white matter. Thus, accumulation half-times of more than 10 min in cortex and 16 min in white matter are taken as signals indicating that simple diffusion instead of active transport governs the accumulation of MG in the respective areas. After steady distribution of MG is achieved, the MG elimination from brain is parallel to the activity in blood; the half-time for both processes is about 50 min and probably reflects renal elimination.

From these time-activity-curves the local perfusion rate (LPR) and local glucose transport rate (LGTR) are calculated simultaneously, as shown in detail in ref. 17 and 29. The results obtained are shown in table 1. These values from normal persons compare favorably with data obtained by others using different methods (5,24,31), and appear to justify our theoretical approach and the assumptions involved in it.

Table 1. Local Glucose transport rate and local perfusion
rate in normal brain

	cortex	white matter	
local glucose transport rate	0.43 - 0.6	0.09 - 0.12	µmol/min g
local perfusion rate	0.08 - 0.98	0.3 - 0.4	ml/min g

In the case demonstrated in fig. 4, values in the region of the primary and associative visual cortex show a parallel reduction of LPR (0.68 ml/min g) and LGTR (0.36 μmol/min g) to 78% of the values of the contralateral side. Thus, in this case, both a metabolic and perfusion response of the visual cortex to the interruption of visual pathways is apparent.

Conclusion

Imbalance between perfusion, transport and metabolism may determine the ultimate damage in ischemic brain disease. Thus, it is desirable to simultaneously determine the local perfusion rate and local glucose transport rate noninvasively. There is good evidence in the data presented that MG is an exellent tracer which, in conjunction with the mathematical model presented, provides the possibility of simultaneously obtaining these data in defined morphological regions.

REFERENCES

1. Raichle ME, Larson KG, Phelps ME, Grubb RL, Welch MJ, Ter-Pogossian MM, Amer. J. Physiol. 228:1936, 1975.

2. Raichle ME, Welch MJ, Grubb RL, Higgins CS, Ter-Pogossian MM, Larson KB, Science 199:986, 1978.

3. Ido T, Wan CN, Casella V, Fowler JS, Wolf AP, Reivich M, Kuhl DE, J. Lab. comp. Radiopharm. 14:175, 1978.

4. Gallagher BM, Fowler JS, Gutterson NI, MacGregor RR, Wan CN, Wolf AP, J. nucl. Med. 19:1154, 1978.

5. Reivich M, Kuhl D, Wolf AP, Greenberg J, Phelps M, Ido T, Casella V, Fowle J, Hoffman E, Alavi A, Som P, Sokoloff L, Circulat. Res. 44:127, 1979.

6. Phelps ME, Huang SC, Hoffman EJ, Selin C, Sokoloff L, Kuhl DE, Ann. Neurol 6:371, 1979.

7. Sokoloff L, Reivich M, Ke-nedy C, Des Rosiers MH, Patlak CS, Pettigrew KD, Sakurada O, Shinohara M, J. Neurochem. 28:897, 1977.

8. Tewson TJ, Welch MJ, Raichle ME, J. nucl. Med. 19:1339, 1978.

9. Goodman MM, Elmaleh DR, Kearfott KJ, Ackerman RH, Hoop B, Brownell GL, Alpert NM, Strauss HW, J. nucl. Med. 22:138, 1981.

10. MacGregor RR, Fowler JS, Wolf AP, Shiue CY, Lade RE, Wan CN, J. nucl. Med. 22:800, 1981.

11. Kloster C, Müller-Platz C, Laufer P, Nucl. Med. Suppl. 17:210, 1980.

12. Kloster G, Müller-Platz C, Laufer P, J. Lab. comp. Radiopharm. 18:855, 198

13. Pardridge WM, Oldendorf WH, Biochim. biophys. Acta 382:377, 1975.

14. Bidder TG, J. Neurochem. 15:867, 1968.

15. Csáky TZ, Wilson JE, Biochim. biophys. Acta 22:185, 1956.

16. Vyska K. Freundlieb C, Höck A, Becker V, Feinendegen LE, Kloster G, Stöckl G, Traupe H, Heiss WD, J. Cer. Blood Flow Metabol. 1, Suppl. 1, S42, 1981.

17. Vyske K, Freundlieb C, Höck A, Becker V, Schmid A, Feinendegen LE, Kloster Stöcklin G, Heiss WD, Radioaktive Isotope in Klinik und Forschung 15:129, 1982.

18. Marazano C, Maziere M, Berger G, Comar D, Int. J. appl. Radiat. Isotopes 28:49, 1977.

19. Laufer P, Kloster G, submitted for publication.

20. Wassenaar W, Tator CH, Batty HP, Cancer Res. 35:785, 1975.

21. Höck A, Freundlieb C, Vyska K, Feinendegen LE, Kloster G, Qaim SM, Stöckli G, Radioaktive Isotope in Klinik und Forschung 14:15, 1980.

22. Heiss WD, Kloster G, Vyska K, Traupe H, Freundlieb C, Becker V, Feinendege LE, Stöcklin G, J. Cer. Blood Flow Metabol. 1, Suppl. 1, S506, 1981.

23. Vyska K, Freundlieb C, Höck A, Becker V, Feinendegen LE, Kloster G, Stöckl G, Traupe H, Heiss WD, Nucl. Med. Suppl. 19, in press, 1982.

24. Kuhl DE, Phelps ME, Kowell AP, Metter EJ, Selin C, Winter J, Ann. Neurol. 8:47, 1980.

25. Betz LA, Gilboe, DD, Brain Res. 65:368, 1974.

26. Gilboe DD, Betz LA, Amer. J. Physiol. 219:774, 1970.

27. Betz LA, Gilboe DD, Yudilevich DL, Drewesir L, Amer. J. Physiol. 225:586, 1973.

28. Whitfield CF, Rames RS, Morgan HE, J. biol. Chem. 249:4181, 1974.

29. Vyska K, Freundlieb C, Höck A, Becker V, Feinendegen LE, Kloster G, Stöcklin G, Heiss WD, Schuier FJ, Thal HU, submitted for publication.

30. Obrist WD, Circ. Rec. 20:124, 1967.

31. Ingvar DA, Cronquist S, Ekberg R, Risberg J, Hoedt-Rasmussen K, Acta Neurol. Scand. 41, Suppl. 14:72, 1965.

THE KINETICS OF [111]IN-DTPA FOR CISTERNOGRAPHY

D.A. TYRRELL

INTRODUCTION

The very delicate nature of the central nervous system means that the neurosurgeon will require as much diagnostic information as possible by non-invasive methods before surgical intervention is contemplated. The technique of radionuclide cisternography can be very useful in such situations to visualize the location, flow and absorption of the cerebrospinal fluid (1,2). A wide variety of radiolabelled agents in both colloidal and soluble form has been proposed for the study of cerebrospinal fluid pathways by isotope cisternography (3). However, only a few of these have proved to be clinically useful. In this paper it will be shown that ^{111}In-DTPA fits the criteria for the ideal cisternographic agent.

Anatomy and physiology of the central nervous system

To enable the properties of the ideal cisternographic agent to be put into perspective it is useful to briefly consider the anatomy and physiology of the fluid spaces within the skull.

The brain and spinal cord are enveloped by three membranes (meninges) named from without inwards the dura mater, the arachnoid mater and the pia mater. The dura mater is a tough fibrous membrane which adheres to the walls of the cranium. Between the dura mater and the closely underlying arachnoid mater is the subdural space. The separation between these membranes permits some movement of the brain in relation to the dura and the skull. The pia mater lines the surface of the brain and spinal cord, exactly following the contours where the arachnoid remains close to the dura. There are gaps between the pia and arachnoid, especially in the regions of large indentations in the surface of the brain. These gaps are called the subarachnoid space and are filled with cerebrospinal fluid (CSF). In certain regions these large fluid filled gaps are known as cisterns.

Inside the brain tissue itself are fluid filled cavities called ventricl
These consist of the two lateral ventricles of the hemispheres connecting wit
the third ventricle in the mid brain region by two small holes called the
foramina of Munro. The third ventricle connects with the fourth ventricle by
a tube called aquaduct of Sylvius. Communication between the ventricular and
subarachnoid fluids is by way of three openings in the fourth ventricle (the
foramen of Magendie and the two foramina of Luschka). The average volume of
the human ventricles is about 23 ml and the total volume of CSF is about 140
so the subarachnoid fluid makes up the larger part.

The major functions of the CSF are as follows:

a. It acts as a fluid cushion for the central nervous system reducing the
   effects of asymmetrical stresses. It obviates large pressure changes durin
   the arterial pulse within the confines of the rigid cranial cavity.

b. Since there is no lymphatic system in the CNS any proteins or other large
   molecular weight substances escaping into the extracellular spaces of the
   brain tissue return to the blood by diffusion into the CSF.

c. The ionic composition of the CSF is such that it contributes to the maintenance of the nerve cells of the brain.

The choroid plexuses are highly vascular regions of the ventricular wall
which are specialized for the formation of CSF. It is now generally agreed th
this is the main if not the exclusive source of the fluid.

The pressure within the CSF remains essentially constant. Thus fluid mus
be removed from the spaces at a similar rate to which it is produced. The
drainage takes place predominantly from the subarachnoid villi or granulation:
These are projections of the subarachnoid space into the various sinuses of
the dura and drainage occurs by osmotic and hydrostatic pressure gradients.

There must be a net flow of cerebrospinal fluid from the site(s) of form
tion to the site of absorption. This depends upon the secretion and absorptio
of CSF proteins. Due to its high osmotic effect protein is absorbed with a
corresponding amount of water, thus creating a bulk flow of CSF. The mixing
and dispersal of fresh choroidal secretion is accelerated by shifts of CSF
resulting from short term changes in the volume of the intracranial blood poo]
due to arterial and venous pressure changes. Full details of CSF formation an
circulation may be found elsewhere (4).

In cisternography radionuclide distribution is mapped after injection int
the subarachnoid space usually into the lumbar region at the base of the spine
The spine is scanned at 1-2 hours to establish the degree of extradural extra-

vasation and to determine whether spinal blocks or abnormalities exist. The
head is then scanned anteriorly and laterally at 2, 6, 24 and 48 hours and the
pattern of distribution within the subarachnoid spaces noted. Cisternography
has found application in the differential diagnosis of hydrocephalus, the
testing of the patency of operative shunts to relieve this condition and the
investigation of pathological CSF leaks.

The ideal cisternographic agent

The anatomical and physiological make-up of the central nervous system
described in the previous section necessitate the ideal cisternographic agent
having a number of specialized properties. In addition the delicate nature of
the investigation places additional concern over aspects of safety. The properties of the ideal agent are listed below.

Table 1. Properties of the ideal cisternographic agent

```
 1. not metabolized in the CSF
 2. lipid insoluble
 3. rapid blood clearance
 4. high rate of liquid diffusion
 5. drainage via arachnoid villi
 6. easily labelled with a gamma emitter
 7. suitable radionuclide properties of the gamma emitter
 8. non irritant
 9. non-antigenic
10. non-toxic
11. non-pyrogenic
12. easily sterilized
```

The CSF possesses a certain enzymatic activity and proteinase activity has
been reported to increase in some disease states. Thus the agent should not be
biochemically cleaved into lower molecular weight fragments which may diffuse
into brain tissue and eventually cause an increase in blood activity. Lipid
insolubility also ensures a minimum of diffusion into surrounding nervous
tissue. The agent, by virtue of low molecular weight or by absence of interaction with the subarachnoid lining should possess a high rate of liquid
diffusion. Once drained via the arachnoid villi blood clearance should be rapid

to minimize background activity and patient radiation dose. Many clinical
conditions require imaging over 24-48 hour period. Thus the radionuclide charac
teristics of the gamma emitter should be such that imaging can be easily carrie
out over this time period. However, an excessively long half life nuclide will
be unsuitable because of the additional radiation dose to the patient.

Factors 8-12 relate to safety aspects and are largely self explanatory.
Non toxicity and non antigenicity of the preparation should be carefully
established as should sterility and lack of pyrogens. The agent should not give
irritation to delicate meningeal membranes after injection into the lumbar subarachnoid space. The osmolarity of the preparation should be carefully controlled in this respect.

^{111}In-DTPA for cisternography

Many radiolabelled agents in both colloidal and soluble form have been
proposed for cisternography (3). Only a few have been proven to be clinically
useful and need be mentioned here. The "traditional" agent became ^{131}I human
serum albumin (HSA) but also in current use are ^{99m}Tc-HSA and ^{99m}Tc-DTPA,
^{169}Yb-DTPA and ^{111}In-DTPA. The half life and safety aspects of the ^{99m}Tc agents
make them unsuitable for general application. ^{131}I HSA may be subject to
proteinase degradation, it is not cleared rapidly from the blood and has less
than ideal radionuclide properties. Thus there remain the ^{169}Yb or ^{111}In comple
es of DTPA. These chelates have been extensively used in cisternographic studie
but there has been concern over the use of ^{169}Yb DTPA from the point of long
term retention in the central nervous system and subsequent high radiation dose
Although claimed safe by some investigators (5-7) there have been several paper
in the literature which have suggested that the agent should not be used (8-10)

At Amersham we have studied the long term clearance of ^{111}In-DTPA and
^{169}Yb-DTPA by whole body counting after intraventricular injection into rats.
The clearance data from these experiments is shown in figs. 1 and 2. The clearance of ^{169}Yb-DTPA was shown to be slower than that of ^{111}In-DTPA and dissection data at 15 days confirmed this. 97% of the ^{111}In-DTPA had been excreted
compared to 93% of the ^{169}Yb-DTPA. Most of the material was excreted through
the kidneys although 6-8% was recovered in the faeces. This was surprising for
DTPA chelates but it was not possible to completely exclude oral ingestion of
small amounts of activity from sites of contamination of the ventral regions
subsequent to the intraventricular injection. Greater tissue retention of ^{169}Yb
DTPA was also observed in autoradiographic studies.

Some in vitro testing of the two agents confirmed the apparently higher in vivo stability of the ^{111}In-DTPA complex. Some dissociation of the ^{169}Yb-DTPA complex was observed by electrophoresis.

These studies together with the clinical reports led us to concentrate our efforts on ^{111}In-DTPA

^{111}In-DTPA is a stable chelate. It is prepared as ^{111}In calcium DTPA to provide excess calcium which will avoid chelation of calcium from the CFS. Bicarbonate buffer is the natural buffer for the CSF, maintaining pH in the range 7.0-7.6. Adverse reactions have been observed after intrathecal administration of material outside this range. Chemical and radionuclidic purity can be carefully controlled and by dispensing the material into flame sealed single dose ampoules and autoclaving the final product maintains the highest safety standards.

A considerable amount of clinical work has now been carried out with ^{111}In-DTPA (11-13). The rate of removal of ^{111}In-DTPA from the CSF has been measured,by Merrick et al,(13) in a series of patients. Typical wash-out curves from the whole body and head are shown in fig. 3. It was shown that in patients examined for 5 days or less the whole body curve could be represented by the sum of 2 exponentials. The mean value of these are given in table 2. In 3 patients examined for a longer period a small third component was detected.

It can be postulated that the fast component is due to renal excretion, the intermediate component reflects diffusion of the chelate from the CFS and the long slow component is due to indium being detached from DTPA and bound to transferrin. No significant long term retention of ^{111}In-DTPA in the central nervous system was observed.

In the light of the animal and clinical data radiation dosimetry estimates have been calculated. It is perhaps useful at this point to compare in detail the most commonly used cisternographic agents. Table 3 summarizes the relevant properties of ^{131}I-HSA, ^{111}In-DTPA and ^{169}Yb-DTPA. In addition to the disadvantages mentioned earlier ^{131}I-HSA suffers from a high radiation dose to the patient. Thus dosage is limited to 100 µCi and poor image quality and hence limited diagnostic value results. In addition it is necessary to block the thyroid to prevent uptake of ^{131}I which has been released in vivo from the HSA. ^{111}In and ^{169}Yb have good nuclear imaging properties making them suitable nuclides for complexing to DTPA for cisternography. However, the longer half life of ^{169}Yb, although offering greater flexibility for off the shelf use by the customer, gives rise to problems in terms of radiation dosimetry. The long

218

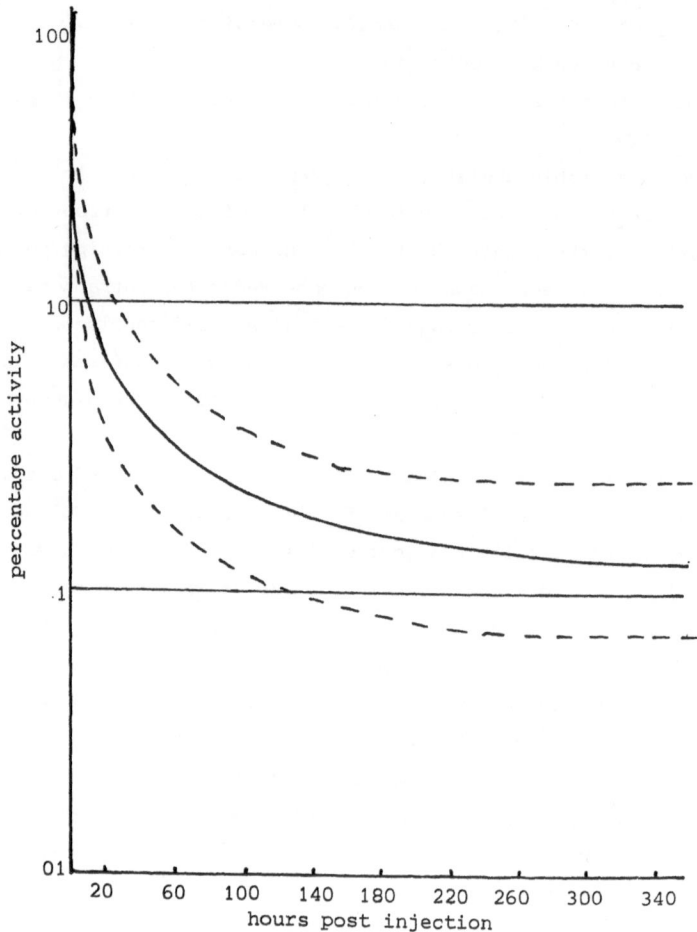

Fig.1. Whole body clearance of ^{111}In-DTPA in the rat
- - - 95% confidence levels.

term retention in the central nervous system observed has led to estimated dos
to the spinal cord of up to 1500 rads / 500 μCi in total CSF block. Such doses
are clearly unacceptable for a nuclear medicine procedure and has greatly
restricted the use of this complex.

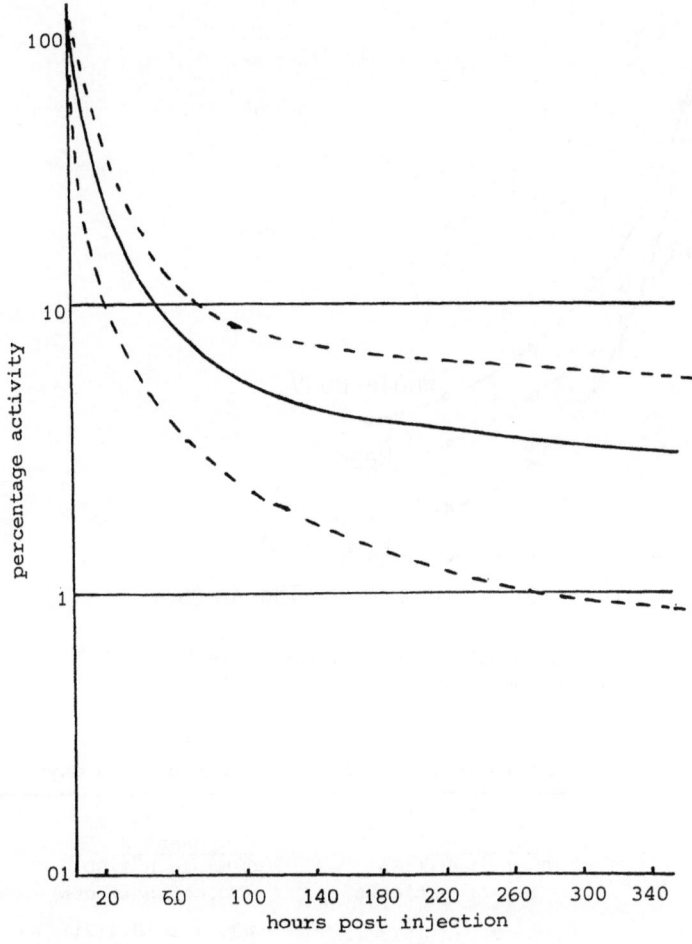

Fig. 2. Whole body clearance of [169]Yb-DTPA in the rat
- - - 95% confidence levels.

Conclusions

^{111}In-DTPA has been shown to meet the criteria listed in table 1 as properties of the ideal cisternographic agents. It is a stable hydrophilic complex
which is not metabolised in the CFS, but which is rapidly cleared by glomerular
filtration from the blood after drainage from the arachnoid villi. [111]In offers
suitable properties for gamma camera scanning and a half life which enables 48
hour scans but which is not long enough to substantially increase radiation
dose. Its nature makes it ideal for production in a safe well-controlled manner.

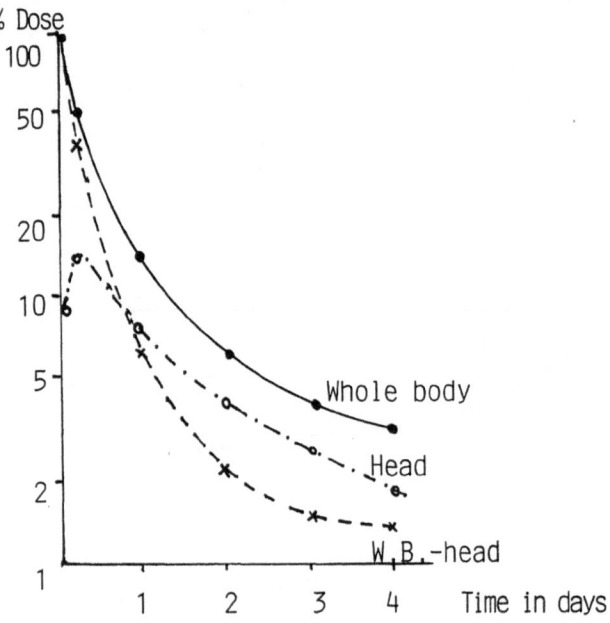

Fig. 3. Typical ^{111}In-DTPA wash-out curve from the whole body, the head and the body (excluding the head).

Table 2a. Clearance of ^{111}In-DTPA in patients studied for up to 5 days

	Component 1 Time in h ± SD (No. of patients)	Component 2 Time in h ± SD (No. of patients)
Whole body	7.8 ± 3.3(16)	43. 1 ± 18.4(21)
Injection site	5.8 ± 1.9(6)	45 ± 9 22 ± 3(4)
Head	not detected	32.5 ± 6 (24)

Table 2b. Patients studied for over 10 days

	Component 1 h ± SD	Component 2 h ± SD	Component 3 h ± SD
Whole body	7.4 ± 3.3	22.8 ± 3.2	209 ± 28
Head		19.4 ± 2.8	236 ± 84

Table 3. Summary of data of commonly used cisternographic agents

	^{131}I-HSA	^{169}Yb-DTPA	^{111}In-DTPA
Physical half life (days)	8.1	32	2.8
Biological half life (hrs)	26	12	10
Useful photon (energy MeV)	0.364	0.177,0.198	0.171,0.247
Useful photons (% disintegration	0.82	0.57	1.83
Whole body dose (rads)	0.17/100μCi	0.069/500μCi	0.039/500μCi
Spinal cord surface dose (rads)	7.1 /100μCi	*8.0 /500μCi	1.9 /500μCi

*Up to 1500R/500μCi for total CSF block

It is non antigenic, non toxic and can be heat sterilized. The simple nature of the complex and its ease of preparation make the introduction of pyrogens unlikely. These features have ensured that ^{111}In-DTPA become the agent of choice for cisterographic studies.

Acknowledgement

Fig. 3. and table 2. are included by kind permission of Dr M. Merrick and the European Journal of Nuclear Medicine.

222

LITERATURE

1. James AE et al. Amer. J. Roentgenol. 110:74, 1970.

2. Holman BL, Davis DO, Progr. nucl. Med. 1:359, 1972.

3. Bell EG et al. in: Cisternography and Hydrocephalus, Harbert JC (ed), 161, 1971.

4. Oldendorf WH, Prog. nucl. Med. 1:336, 1972.

5. Wagner HN et al. Radiology, 95:121, 1970.

6. Deland FH, J. nucl. Med. 14:93, 1973.

7. Deland FH, J. nucl. Med. 12:683, 1971.

8. Barbizet J et al. Nouv. Presse. Med. 1:2899, 1972.

9. Alazraki N et al. J. nucl. Med. 15:643, 1974.

10. Christiansen K, Aust. Radiol. 19:25, 1975.

11. Goodwin DA et al. Radiology, 108:91, 1973.

12. Rhodes BA, Radiology, 119:749, 1976.

13. Merrick MV et al. Eur. J. nucl. Med. 3:105, 1978.

COMPLICATIONS AFTER INTRATHECAL ADMINISTRATION OF Tc^{99m} DTPA

A. VERBRUGGEN, M. de ROO, P. DEWIT, P. GUELINCKX, R. DOM

INTRODUCTION

DTPA labelled with ^{111}In is the radiopharmaceutical with the most suitable properties for isotope cisternography (1,2). DTPA labelled with Tc^{99m} is a valuable alternative for cases not requiring scans later than 24 hours after injection as reported by Som and co-workers in 1972 (3) and later on by other authors (4,5). The advantages and disadvantages of these two tracer substances in terms of their suitability as radiopharmaceutical for cisternographic scinti-

TABLE I: COMPARISON OF ^{111}In-DTPA and ^{99m}Tc-DTPA FOR CISTERNOGRAPHY

^{111}In-DTPA	^{99m}Tc-DTPA
Ideal physical properties	Physical T1/2 sufficient in most cases
Delayed scans possible	Delayed scans (> 24 h) not possible
Purity checked by manufacturer	Purity partly dependent on preparation in the hospital
Not toxic	Possibly toxic
Radiation dose to spinal cord (7,8)	
3.8 mrad/mCi	0.21 mrad/mCi
Moderate resolution for 0.5 mCi	Excellent resolution for 5-7 mCi
Available once a week	Available all the time
Expensive	Inexpensive

TABLE II: CASES WITH SIDE EFFECTS AFTER INTRATHECAL ADMINISTRA⌐
OF ^{99m}Tc-DTPA (type A)

CLINICAL HISTORY

Day 0: (intrathecal injection) no symptoms

Day 1: fever (1), sciatic neuritis pain (2)

Day 5: - retention of urine and feces (1,2)

$\qquad$ (Hypoesthesia: - moderate in L_2 - L_3 (1)

$\qquad$ - $\qquad$ { $\qquad\qquad\quad$ - pronounced in S_2 - S_4 (1,2)

$\qquad$ (Anesthesia in S_4 - S_5 (saddle anesthesia) (1,2)

$\qquad$ - weakness of m. iliopsoas (L_2 - L_3)

$\qquad\qquad\qquad\qquad$ mmi. glutei (L_5 - S_2)

9 $\qquad\qquad\qquad\quad$ m. quadriceps(L_2 - L_4)

Day 12: - saddle anesthesia

$\qquad$ - fecal and urinary incontinence

After one year symptoms unchanged

(1) patient 1

(2) patient 2

graphy are presented in table I.

Whereas with ^{111}In-DTPA scintigrams can be made up to 72 hours after injection, the short physical half-life of Tc^{99m}-DTPA does not permit scans lat⌐
than 24 hours after injection, but in most cases this is sufficient to make t]
diagnosis. According to Bell et al (6), only 10% of the patients submitted fo:
isotope cisternography need to be studied beyond 24 hours. They routinely
perform the study initially with a Tc^{99m} labelled compound and then repeat wit
^{111}In-DTPA, when necessary.

The purity of Tc^{99m}-DTPA cannot be guaranteed by any manufacturer, as it
depends not only on the purity of the cold DTPA kit and of the Tc^{99m}-eluate, k
also on the techniques used by radiopharmacist or technician in the hospital.
^{111}In-DTPA has proven to be a safe radiopharmaceutical for cisternography whe⌐
as the possible toxicity of Tc^{99m}-DTPA when injected into the cerebrospinal
fluid may present a serious restriction to its use.

The arguments in favour of Tc^{99m}-DTPA are well known: the low radiation dose permits the administration of a high activity preparation, producing images with an excellent resolution. It is also readily available at very low cost, whereas it can take up to ten days before the more expensive ^{111}In-DTPA is available.

We began to use Tc^{99m}-DTPA for cisternography a few years ago because of its attractive properties, the positive literature reports and in view of the urgency with which neurologists often require results. At the time, we were routinely using a Tc^{99m}-DTPA preparation reconstituted from a cold DTPA kit from a commercial source for brain and kidney scintigraphy. Some authors had reported using the same preparation for cisternography, our cisternoscintigraphic explorations were also performed after injection of this tracer substance. After reconstruction with 15 mCi Tc^{99m}-eluate in 2 ml, we injected half the content of the vial containing about 7,5 mCi of Tc^{99m} via an intralumbar punction at L_3-L_4. Excellent scintigrams were obtained and a valuable diagnosis was made in our first 15 cases.

Adverse reactions after intrathecal injection of Tc^{99m}-DTPA

Two of the first 15 patients developed adverse neurological reactions. The first case (patient 1) was a 60 year old female suspected of normal pressure hydrocephaly. Isotope cisternography showed abnormal ventricle filling still present at 24 hours. The second case (patient 2) was a 50 year old man with a pituitary adenoma who developed rhinorrhea, probably through the sinus sphenoidalis. The presence of cisternal fluid in the rhinopharynx was detected by isotope cisternography.

The clinical progress of these 2 patients was very similar and can be summarized as shown in table II. On the day of the intrathecal injection no complaints were noted. On the next day, 1 patient developed fever, and the other complained of sciatic neuritis pain. From day 5 to 9 there was urinary and fecal retention, moderate hypoesthesia in L_1-L_3, pronounced hypoesthesia in S_2-S_3, and complete anaesthesia in S_3-S_5, the so-called saddle anaesthesia. There was also weakness of some hip and thigh muscles. Two weeks after the intrathecal injection the patients complained of fecal and urinary incontinence, but the only sensory disturbance that remained was saddle anaesthesia. At a check-up one year later, these symptoms were still present without any noticeable change.

During a retrospective investigation of the whole matter, we were informed of other cases of side-effects after the intrathecal injection of the same Tc^{99m}-

DTPA preparation. In one clinic, a patient was reported to have manifested the same signs of the cauda equina syndrome as did our 2 patients. In addition to other cases of benign complications such as headache and fever, there were also several mentions of severe signs of meningitis, meningo encephalitis, and meningo myelitis, and 1 patient died with numerous non-specified neurological symptoms.

TABLE III: COMPOSITION OF DTPA KITS OF DIFFERENT SOURCES

MANUFACTURER	mg CaNa$_3$ DTPA	mg SnCl$_2$	pH
A	not indicated *	not indicated*	not indicate
B	9.1	0.38	4 - 6.5
C	25	0.25	4
D	9.5	0.5	4
E	5	0.45	4
F	10	0.5	4

*Package insert
.... reagent for the single-step instant preparation of the pure chelate Tc^{99m}-Sn-DTPA (diethylenetriamine-pentaacetic acid). It contains neither iron nor ascorbate.
Information provided by manufacturer A
H$_5$DTPA   24   mg
SnCl$_2$.2H$_2$O   3.6 mg
pH   7 ± 0.5

From another clinic we were informed of 3 patients with an appilic syndrome after suboccipital injection of Tc^{99m}-DTPA from the same manufacturer. One of them also showed signs of a conus lesion. The first of these patients died; the second was saved, but presented severe and persistent neurological deficits; the third one recovered uneventfully.

The origin of the adverse reactions

It seemed to us highly probably that the adverse reactions in these patients had been provoked by one or more ingredients of the DTPA preparation used. We looked for the composition of the cold DTPA kit of the manufacturer, but no information about the identity or quantity of the kit ingredients could be found on the package insert or the vial label. The composition of all the other DTPA kits commercially available in our country at that time was clearly described (table III).

All these preparations contained between 5 and 25 mg of DTPA in the form of its calcium trisodium salt and up to 0.5 mg of stannous chloride. The pH of these preparations was indicated to be about 4. The manufacturer informed us that his cold DTPA kits contained per vial, 24 mg DTPA in acid form, thus not as a calcium trisodium salt, and a surprisingly high amount of stannous chloride, 7 to 14 times higher than in the other comparable DTPA kits. As the reconstituted DTPA preparation has a pH of 7, the DTPA is present in the form of its trisodium salt. The schematic structure of trisodium DTPA and of calcium trisodium DTPA is represented in table IV. A very important difference between the two chemical

TABLE IV.   STRUCTURE OF H_2Na_3 DTPA AND OF $CaNa_3$ DTPA

H_2 Na_3 DTPA

$$
\begin{array}{c}
HOOC - CH_2 \\
HOOC - CH_2
\end{array} N - CH_2 - CH_2 - \underset{\underset{COONa}{\overset{|}{CH_2}}}{N} - CH_2 - CH_2 - N \begin{array}{c} CH_2 - COO\ Na \\ CH_2 - COO\ Na \end{array}
$$

Ca Na_3 DTPA

$$
Ca \begin{array}{c}
^{..}OOC - CH_2 \\
^{..}OOC - CH_2
\end{array} N - CH_2 - CH_2 - \underset{\underset{COONa}{\overset{|}{CH_2}}}{N} - CH_2 - CH_2 - N \begin{array}{c} CH_2 - COO\ Na \\ CH_2 - COO\ Na \end{array}
$$

forms of DTPA is that trisodium DTPA is able to strongly complex all kinds of metallic ions, such as Ca, Mg, Tc and In, whereas calcium trisodium DTPA can bind Tc and In but not Ca or Mg.

As shown in table V hydrogen ions are liberated when Ca or Mg ions are complexed by trisodium DTPA which causes both a diminution of the concentration of free Ca and Mg ions and a local drop of the pH. From our knowledge of the identity and the quantity of the ingredients in the DTPA kit of our manufacturer

TABLE V.   INTERACTION OF H_2Na_3 DTPA AND METAL IONS

$$H_2Na_3DTPA + \begin{matrix} Ca^{++} \\ Mg^{++} \end{matrix} \rightleftharpoons \begin{matrix} CaNa_3\ DTPA \\ MgNa_3\ DTPA \end{matrix} + 2H^+$$

- CBS FLUID: Ca^{++} = 2.28 mEq/ml

            Mg^{++} = 2.23 mEq/ml

       METAL IONS   4.51 mEq/ml

and taking into account the composition of the cerebrospinal fluid (9), we can summarize the alterations in the cerebrospinal fluid provoked by intrathecal injection of half the content of a vial of this DTPA preparation as follows:
- 5 ml of cerebrospinal fluid are completely depleted of Ca and Mg ions. One
  can assume that after a very slow intrathecal injection of 1 ml of a prepara
  tion, this injected solution is first mixed with no more than about 5 ml of
  the cerebrospinal fluid. If the cerebrospinal fluid at the site of injection
  is moving slowly, this situation may persist for a relatively long period,
  leaving the nerves in contact with a Ca-free or Ca-poor medium.
- At the site of injection the pH drops from the normal 7.35 to about 6.7 which
  we determined experimentally.
- The nerves at the injection site are exposed to the possible chemical toxici
  of 12 mg DTPA and of the tin present in 1.8 mg stannous chloride. The presen
  of tin is not without importance as some tin compounds are known to be highl
  neurotoxic and produce symptoms comparable to those observed in our patients
  (10).
- Impurities in the Tc^{99m}-eluate may also interact with the normal nerve
  function. However, we did not entertain this possibility further as the orig
  of the side-effects, because no adverse reactions in 85 cisternographies wit
  another type of Tc^{99m}-DTPA were observed.

Pharmacological study

In order to determine which of these reactions, namely the depletion of C and Mg ions or the drop of the pH to an abnormally low value, or the chemical toxicity of the ingredients of the DTPA kit, had been responsible for the

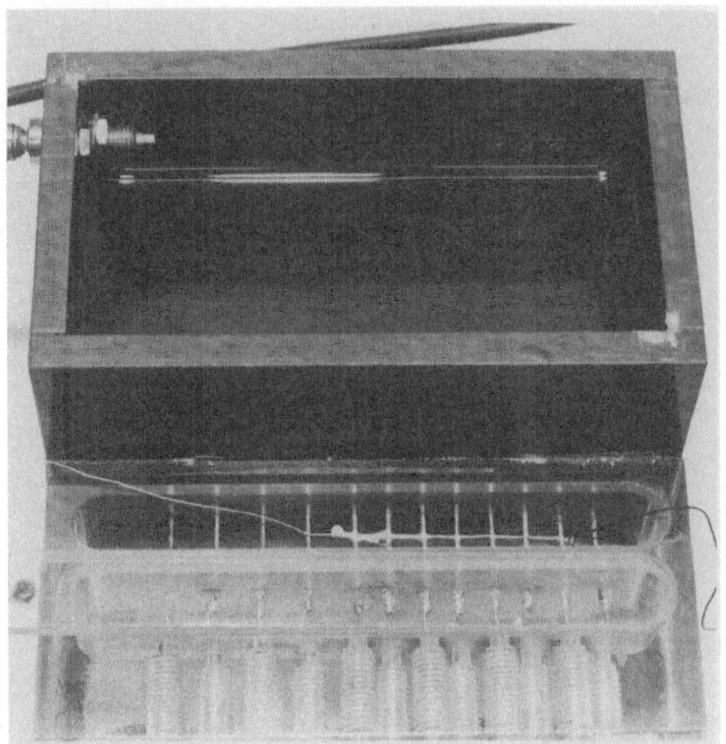

Fig. 1. Organ bath with electrodes for the stimulation of the nerve and the determination of the extracellular potential changes.

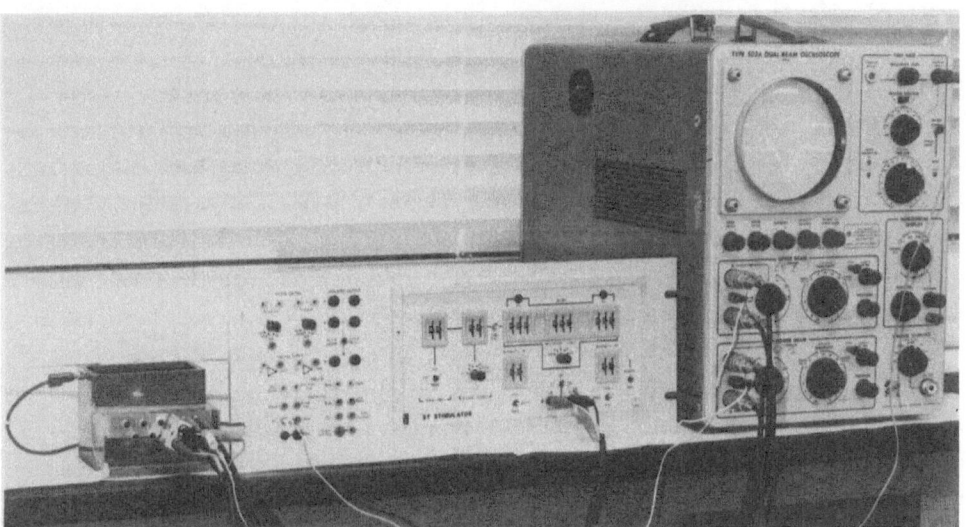

Fig. 2. Experimental set-up for investigation of the pulse conduction in isolated nerves. From left to right: organ bath, stimulator, oscilloscope.

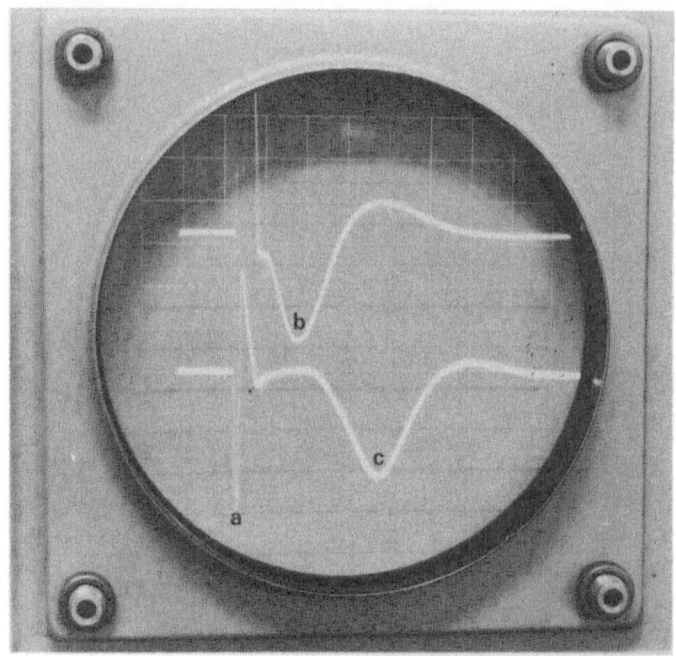

Fig. 3. Extracellular potential changes in isolated rat ischiatic nerve on oscilloscope display: a) artefact of stimulation; b-c) extracellular potentia at first (b) and second (c) pair of measuring electrodes.

observed adverse reactions, a pharmacological study was carried out with expe ments on rabbits in vivo. The results were disappointing as it was not possib to establish structural or functional modifications in the nerves to which stannous DTPA had been applied.

Experiments on isolated ischiatic nerves of rats yielded more useful in-formation. The isolated ischiatic nerves were suspended in a solution with th same ionic composition as the cerebrospinal fluid (9). Different amounts of stannous DTPA, DTPA alone in both chemical forms, tin, or hydrogen ions were added to lower the pH. After different time intervals, the nerves were taken of the solution and placed on a set of electrodes as shown in fig. 1.

The nerve was than electrically stimulated by the first pair of electrod The conduction of the action potential was analyzed by registration of the ext cellular potential changes at the two following electrode pairs. Fig. 2 shows the complete experimental construction. On the display (fig. 3) after a brief artefact due to stimulation the registration of the extracellular potential a the first and second pair of measuring electrodes can be seen.

TABLE VI: EFFECTS OF STANNOUS DTPA, SN OR pH ON PULSE CONDUCTION

IN ISOLATED RAT ISCHIATIC NERVE

NERVE IN CONTACT WITH	PULSE CONDUCTION

Sn-H$_2$Na$_3$ DTPA
     DTPA   5   mEq/l[*]
     Sn   0.75 mEq/l[*]
	Blocked after 15 h

H$_2$Na$_3$ DTPA   2.5   mEq/l[+]
             5   mEq/l
             10   mEq/l
             20   mEq/l
	Reduced after 15 h
	 Blocked after 15 h
	 Blocked after 5 h
	 Blocked after 2 h

CaNa$_3$ DTPA 20 mEq/l	Normal

SnCl$_2$
 Sn-CaNa$_3$DTPA   3   mEq/l
            1.5   mEq/l
            0.75 mEq/l[*]
	- (precipitation of Sn-compound)
	 Reduced but reversible
	 Normal
	 Normal

CBS fluid pH 6.7 [*]	Normal

[*]situation after injection of 1/2 vial Tc^{99m}-DTPA in 5 ml CBS fluid.

[+]concentration metal ions in CBS fluid = 4.5 mEq/l.

Table VI summarizes the results of these experiments. A concentration of stannous DTPA, comparable to the situation in the cerebrospinal fluid after the injection of half the content of a vial Tc^{99m}-DTPA of our manufacturer in 5 ml cerebrospinal fluid, completely blocks pulse condition after 15 hours. The same concentration of trisodium DTPA alone provokes the same effect. A lower concentration of trisodium DTPA, which leaves some Ca and Mg ions in the solution, affects the nerve function but does not destroy it. A higher concentration of trisodium DTPA than necessary for the complete sequestration of the Ca and Mg

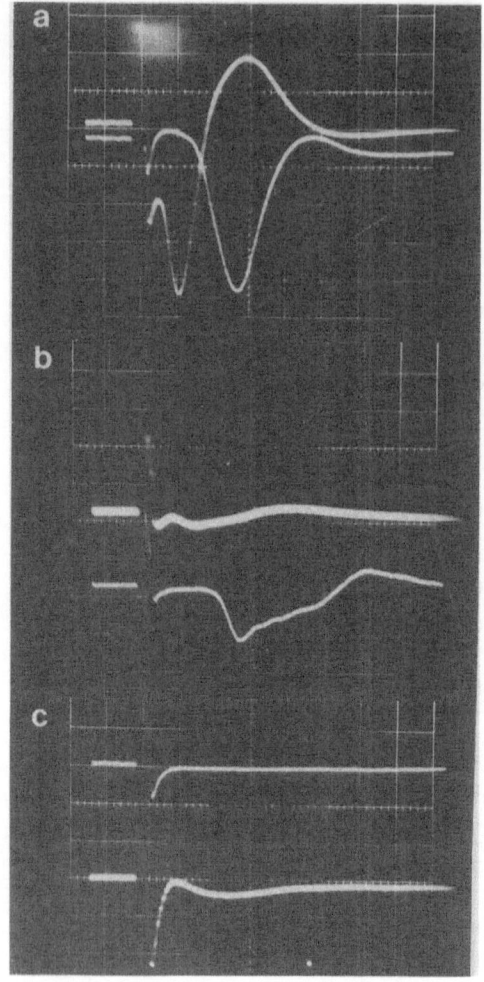

Fig. 4. Effect of trisodium DTPA (5 mEq/l) on pulse conduction in isolated rat ischiatic nerve. Horizontal scale: 1 division = 0.5 msec. Vertical scale: 1 division = 1 mV. a. Before contact with Na_3DTPA. b. After 4 hours contact. c. After 10 hours contact.

ions blocks the pulse conduction much earlier.

Fig. 4 illustrates what happens when the nerve function is affected by tr sodium DTPA 5 mEq/l. After a few hours the conduction velocity, measured as th ratio of the distance between the first and second electrode pair to the diffe ence in time to peak is not greatly affected. However, the extracellular negat peaks are smaller and much wider suggesting that most but not all fibres in th

multifibre bundle have markedly decreased conduction velocity. After a contact
of 10 hours, the pulse signal has completely disppeared.

It is interesting to note that Ca DTPA, even in very high concentrations,
does not affect the nerve function at all, nor does a pH drop from 7.35 to 6.7.
It was not possible to study the effect of stannous chloride alone, as its
addition to the solution resulted in immediate precipitation. Therefore, we had
to complex tin, and we used for this purpose CaNa$_2$DTPA, which as we had previously demonstrated is harmless to the nerve. Only high concentrations of stannous
DTPA affect the nerve function, and this effect appeared to be readily reversible,
unlike that of trisodium DTPA. From these experiments, we concluded that the
complexing properties of trisodium DTPA were responsible for the observed modifications in the nerve function.

Conclusions
- The adverse reactions following intrathecaal application of Tc^{99m}-DTPA from our
  manufacturer were apparently provoked by the sequestration of Ca and Mg ions
  in the cerebrospinal fluid at the site of injection.
- Since nerve membrane permeability is modified by a low concentration of Ca
  ions, a direct chemical toxicity of DTPA and tin is not excluded. Our observation that trisodium DTPA in a concentration higher than necessary for the
  complete sequestration of the Ca and Mg ions affects the nerve function earlier, depending on the concentration could be interpreted in this way.
- Stannous DTPA can affect nerve function at very high concentrations, but this
  effect is reversible by the removal of the tin compound.

Some more general remarks are also in order:
- Radiopharmaceuticals, despite their low content of ingredients, may provoke
  adverse reactions and do not merit their reputation of absolute safety.
- It is absolutely necessary that the composition of the kits for labelling with
  Tc^{99m} should be indicated on the package insert and/or on the vial label.
- From our further experience with Tc^{99m}-DTPA in cisternographic scintigraphy,
  we have learned that Tc^{99m}-DTPA prepared from a kit containing calcium trisodium DTPA and a low content of stannous chloride can safely be used for
  cisternography. We now use a kit containing 9.1 mg CaNa$_3$ DTPA and 0.45 mg
  SnCl$_2$; 75 mCi of Tc^{99m}-eluate is added accepticaly in 5 ml and after 15 min
  the pH is adjuncted to 7 with sterile NaOH(0.05 normal) the required volume of
  which we previously determined in another vial of the same batch. After

quality control, we inject 5-7 mCi of this preparation, which contains at mo
one tenth of the content of the preparation. In 85 cisternographies with thi
Tc^{99m}-DTPA preparation, we have observed no adverse reactions.

- However, some precautions are absolutely necessary. The preparation has to b
formulated by or under the supervision of a radiopharmacist or radiochemist
familiar with sterility, pyrogenicity and chemical toxicity. The Tc^{99m}-eluat
should be freshly eluted from a generator, in use no longer than three days.
In this way the risk of pyrogens is minimized as every manufacturer of Tc^{99m}
generators quarantees the absence of pyrogens at the moment of delivery.
Finally, a strict aseptic procedure must be adhered to.

Acknowledgements

The authors wish to thank Dr J. Vereecke for his helpful discussions and
advice, Mrs. M. Hoogmartens for expert technical assistance in the animal expe
iments, and Mrs. M.J. Vangoetsenhoven for graciously typing the text.

REFERENCES

1. Matin P, Goodwin DA, Cerebrospinal fluid scanning with [111]In. J. nucl. Med. 12:668, 1971.

2. Hosain F, Phil D, Som P, Chelated [111]In: an ideal radiopharmaceutical for cisternography. Brit. J. Radiol. 45:677, 1972.

3. Som P, Hosain F, Wagner HN jr, Scheffel U, Cisternography with chelated complex of 99m-TC. J. nucl. Med. 13:551, 1972.

4. Oberson R, La myéloscintigraphie. Schweiz. med. Wschr. 36:1237, 1974.

5. Oberson R, Détection des fuites de liquide céphalorachidien par gammacisternographie. Neuro-chirurgie 22:397, 1976.

6. Bell EG, Maher B, McAfee JG, Subramanian G, Radiopharmaceuticals for gamma cisternography. In: Radiopharmaceuticals, Subramanian G et al. (eds) Society of Nuclear Medicine, New York, 1975, p. 390.

7. Goodwin DA, Sunberg MW, Diamanti CI, Meares CF, III-In-labeled radiopharmaceuticals and their clinical use. In: Radiopharmaceuticals, Subramanian G et al. (eds) Society of Nuclear Medicine, New York, 1975, p. 80.

8. Yano Y, Radionuclide Generators: current and futur applications in nuclear medicine. In: Radiopharmaceuticals, Subramanian G et al. (eds) Society of Nuclear Medicine, New York, 1975, p. 237.

9. Tables Scientifiques, 7 ième édition, Ciba Geigy, Bâle, p. 647, 1972.

10. HP "Stalinon": a therapeutic disaster. Brit. med. J. p. 515, 1958.

EIN NEUES RADIOPHARMAKON-MODELL FÜR DIE AUGENTUMORSZINTIGRAPHIE

G. LIMOURIS, M. TSIROU

EINLEITUNG

Bislang hat in der Ophtalmologie die Augenszintigraphie als Routinemethode
für die klinische Diagnostik noch keinen Eingang gefunden. Dies ist einmal darauf
zurückzuführen, dass bisher noch kein geeignetes γ-e-mittierendes Radionuklid
entwickelt wurde, welches sich selektiv im Auge konzentriert, zun anderen darauf,
dass das Sehorgan vom Knochenschutz umgeben ist, welcher seine Szintigraphie
erschwert. Wie in der Tabelle 1 dargestellt ist, wurden bis heute viele radioaktive Substanzen für die Augenszintigraphie geprüft mit mehr oder weniger Erfolg.

·Tabelle I

Pharmakon	Markierungsnuklid
Na-Phosphat	P^{32}
Galliumzitrat	G^{67}
Jodoquinolin	I^{125}
Jodochloroquin	I^{131}
4.3 Dimethylamino-propylamino-7-iodoquinolin	I^{123}
Pertechnetat	Tc^{99m}
Tris-aminomethan	Pb^{203}

Vorliegende Arbeit befasst sich mit der Möglichkeit der Augentumorszintigraphie,
nach Applikation eines mit zwei Radionukliden markierten Substanz-Modells, dieses
von Fluoreszein. Als Laboratoriummodell ist das Melanom des menslichen Auges er-
wähnt.

Unser radioaktives Substanzmodell besteht aus zwei Teilen (Fig. 1):
- dem Pharmakon
- den zwei Markierungsnukliden.
Als Pharmakon wird Fluoreszeinsodium gewält und als Markierungsnuklid ein beta-

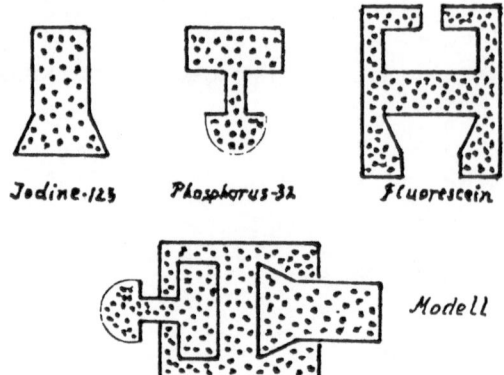

Fig. 1.

emittierendes, nämlich Phosphor-32 und ein gamma-emittierendes und zwar Jod-123

Fluoreszein ($C_{20}H_{12}O_5$). Es handelt sich um einen gelbroten Farbstoff desse verdünnte Lösung stark grün fluoresziert, in einem Spektralbereich zwischen 500 - 530 nm. Diese Substanz ist in der diagnostischen Ophtalmologie als Fluors zeinsodium (Salz) sehr bekannt, da es routinenmässig für die Fluorangiographie intravenös injeziert wird. Es ist auch als Resorcinophtalein bekannt.

Phosphor-32. Die vom Augenmelanom Phosphor-32 Aufnahme ist der Spiegel der Phosphateioneninkorporation im DNA und RNA der neuentstehenden Nuklearsäuren de Zellkernes. Da diese wichtige metabolische Funktion von dieser bösartigen Vermehrung abhängt, läuft der Wert der Phosphor-32-Aufnahme parallel zur bös- artigen Vergrösserung. Dieses Phosphor-32-Benehmen ist typisch, fast einzig für Markierungsnuklid für die Tumorlokalisation (1,2). Die Tendenz der Phosphorione eine höhere Konzentration im bösartigen als im normalen Geweben zu zeigen, er- klärt ihre längere Verhaltung vom Tumor, ein charakteristisches Merkmal von wichtiger klinischer Bedeutung. Phosphor-32 emittiert ausschliesslich beta- strahlen (1.71 MeV) mit einer Halbwertszeit vom 14.3 Tagen.

Jod-123. Dieses im Zyklotron produzierbare Radionuklid, wurde in den letzt Jahren in der Nuklearmedizin eingeführt. Seine Halbwertszeit von 13.3 h und seine Gammaemission (0.59 MeV, 84%) macht es zum idealsten Radiojod bis heute.

Methode.

Der Nachweis von malignen Geschwülsten mit radioaktiv markierten Substanze ist seit langer Zeit Gegenstand ausgedehnter klinischexperimenteller Untersuch- ungen gewesen. Trotz vieler optimistischer Berichte (3,4,5) steht auch heute kein tumorspezifisches Radiopharmakon der Nuklearmedizin zur Verfügung, offenba

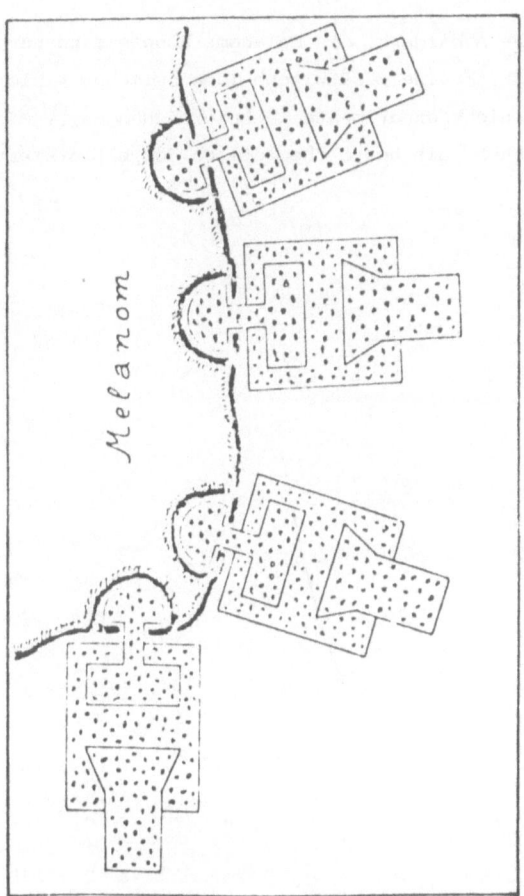

Fig. 2.

weil sich der Tumorstoffwechsel nur gering von dem des normalen Gewebes unter-
scheidet. Die Entwicklung des nuklearmedizinischen Tumornachweises ist bestimmt
keinesfalls abgeschlossen und gute Ergebnisse sind in der Zukunft zu erwarten.

Melanome des Augen sind Tumoren mit erhöhtem speziellen Stoffwechsel in Ab-
hängigkeit zur Wachstumsrate (DNA-Synthese) mit grösser als 25% erhöhter Phos-
phoraufnahme im Vergleich zur Umgebung.

Basierend auf der Affinität des Phosphors-32 zu den Melanomen, wird das
damit markierte Fluoreszein zum Tumor mitgeschleppt. Da aber auch im Fluores-
zeinmolekül Jod-123 inkorporiert ist, könnte man durch die Eigenschaft dieses
Gammastrahlenemittierenden Radionuklides, den lokalisatorischen Nachweis der in-
korporierten Radioaktivität mittels beweglicher (Scanner) oder feststehender
(Gamma-Kamera) Szintigraphiegeräte (siehe Fig. 2) erbringen. Eine gute und

genaue szintigraphische Abbildung des Melanoms könnte dann hergestellt werden Diese Arbeit hat als Zweck eine zusätzliche Idee zwischen viele andere zu werf und Gedanken und vielleicht experimentelle Untersuchungen, für die mögliche Applikation einer solchen, bis heute theoretisch doppeltmarkierten Substanz zu gebären.

LITERATUR

1. Homburger F, Fishman WH, The Physiopathology of Cancer, Hoeber Harper, 1953, p. 584.

2. O'Rourke J, Nuclear Ophtalmology, Saunders Comp. Ltd. London-Philadelphia-Toronto, 1976.

3. z. Winkel K, Die diagnostische Bedeutung radioaktiver Isotope für die Ophtalmologie. Ber. dtsch. ophtal. Ges. 76:251, Heidelberg, 1979.

4. Beckslaff H, Dausch D, Stoeppler L, Hundeshagen H, Safi N, Blanquet P, Gamma-Kamera, Funktionsszintigraphie zum Nachweis intraokularer Veränderungen. Technisches Konzept und klinische Beispiele. Ber. dtsch. ophtal. Ges. 76:321, Heidelberg, 1979.

5. Bockslaff H, Dausch D, Stoeppler L, Honegger H, Hundeshagen H, Gamma-Szintigraphie mit einem Doppel-Lochblenden-Kollimator zum nichtinvasiven Nachweis intraokularer Veränderungen. Ber. dtsch. ophtal. Ges. 76:303, Heidelberg, 1979.

MATHEMATICS IN RADIOPHARMACOLOGY: A NECESSARY SYMBIOSIS

G. LIMOURIS, G. YANNIKAKIS

INTRODUCTION

"How far even then mathematics will suffice to describe and explain the fabric of the body, no man can foresee".

With these words D'Arcy Wentworth Thompson in his book "On Growth and Form" in the year 1917 (1) expressed the importance of mathematics to express human-organ function. It is possible to consider these words as prophetic if, as scientists concerned with the actual progress of medical science, we compare to-day with that period. It is indisputable that this progress is primarily due to the vast evolution of a technology which is based upon mathematical thought and creativity.

In the field of radiopharmacology, the biodistribution of radiopharma-ceuticals can be reduced to mathematical symbols for the easier study of their characteristics in order to evaluate their properties. A number of mathematical relationships related to radiotracer-kinetics clearly indicate the necessity and value of a skeptical mathematical method. These mathematical relationships bind chemistry, physiology, pharmacology and medicine to one another in the common pursuit of the study of tracer-kinetics. The term radiopharmaceutical may be defined as a radio-indicator which emits penetrating radiation and is used specifically for diagnostic and some times for therapeutic purposes.

The pharmaco-kinetics of radiopharmaceuticals were studied in particular relation to the calculation of radiation doses delivered to organs and whole body. Half-life, radiation decay, decay factors, transient equilibrium, clear-ance, calculated dose are nomen terminologies utilized in the field of radio-tracer kinetics. They reflect the biological effect of radiopharmaceuticals and are to-day expressed as mathematical formulations.

Half-life

The length of time a radionuclide is present in an organ is determined by (a) the effective half-life ($T\frac{1}{2}$ eff)- the physical half-life ($T\frac{1}{2}$ phy) and (b)

$$\tfrac{1}{2}N_o = N_o \, e^{-\lambda T_{\frac{1}{2}}} \;\rightarrow\; T_{\frac{1}{2}} = \frac{\ln 2}{\lambda} = \frac{0.693}{\lambda}$$

$$T_{\frac{1}{2}} eff = \frac{(T_{\frac{1}{2}} \; bio) \times (T_{\frac{1}{2}} \; phy)}{T_{\frac{1}{2}} \; bio + T_{\frac{1}{2}} \; phy}$$

Fig. 1.

the biological half-life ($T_{\frac{1}{2}}$ bio), and can be illustrated by the following mathematical formulas as expressed in fig. 1.

Decay of radioactivity - transient equilibrium (2)

Mathematically radioactive decay is described in terms of probabilities ε average decay rates as shown in fig. 2. The average decay rate, expressed by

(1) $\Delta N/\Delta t = -\lambda N$

(2) $\tau = 1/\lambda$

(3) $DF = (\tfrac{1}{2})^n (1-\tfrac{1}{2}f)$

(4) $A_t(t) = A_1(0) \, e^{-0.693t/T_{\frac{1}{2},1}} +$

   $A_2(0) \, e^{-0.693t/T_{\frac{1}{2},2}} + \ldots\ldots$

   $dN_p/dt = -\lambda_p N_p$

   $dN_d/dt = -\lambda_d N_d + \lambda_p N_n$

(5) $N_d(t) = N_p(0) \dfrac{\lambda d}{\lambda d - \lambda p} (e^{-\lambda_p t} - e^{-\lambda_d t}) + N_d(0) e^{-\lambda_d t}$

   $A_d(t) = A_p(0) \dfrac{\lambda d}{\lambda d - \lambda p} (e^{-\lambda_p t} - e^{-\lambda d^t}) + A_d(0) e^{-\lambda_d t}$

(6) $A_d(A_p = T_p/(T_p - T_d)$

Fig. 2.

formula (1), the average time τ by formula (2), the approximate method for the accurate estimation of the decay factor, by formula (3), the equation for the estimation of the decay of a mixed radionuclide sample in formula (4), the equation by a simple parent-daughter mixture (named Bateman equation), by formula (5) and the calculation of the transient equilibrium of daughter and parent activity by formula (6).

Clearance

For calculating the volume of plasma in each minute from which all activity might have been cleared the following expression is used:

$$\text{CLEARANCE} = \frac{U \, V}{\int_{t_1}^{t2} Pdt}$$

Calculated dose (3)

To calculate the internal radiation dose, the classical mathematical expressions were developed by Hine and Brownell in 1958, for beta and gamma emitters as expressed by formulas (1) and (2) in fig. 3. Similar expressions werd developed by Loevinger and Berman in 1968, Smit (1968), Snyder (1969), and Berger (1971)

(1)	$D\beta(\infty)$	$= 73.8 \, \bar{E}\beta\Sigma_i C_i T_i$ rads
(2)	$D\gamma(\infty)$	$= 0.036 \, \rho\bar{\Gamma}\bar{g}\Sigma_i C_i T_i$ roentgens
(3)	$|D|$	$= f \, (x,y,z,t)$
(4)	Y	$= Ae^{-at} + Be^{-\beta t} + Ce^{-\gamma t}$

Fig. 3.

Radionuclide distribution (4)

Radionuclide distribution has been studied in order to compute the radiation dose within organs which are not the target organ. The calculation is accomplishe using a simple matrix notation, expressed by formula (3) in fig. 3. The symbol D in matrix notation is used for the word distribution. Since a radiopharmaceutical can be considered as a signal generator, the above matrix has dimensions of the three spatial co-ordinates (x,y,z) and the forth dimension of time (t). Thus the images obtained in nuclear medicine are recorded in only one spatial plane (x,y) at one time (t). The three-dimensional information is obtained by making images

from different points of view. Since the images obtained are also matrices, t
allows the mathematical representation of the image to the total data base, i
other words the biodistribution. The equation expressed by formula (4) descri
radioactivity in blood against time, representing the kinetics of distributio

In conclusion I would like to related a story of a young mathematics
instructor refered to in a mathematics book "Mathematical methods in the phys
sciences" (5), who asked an older professor: "What do you say when you are ask
about the practical applications of some mathematical topic?". His colleague
replied: "I tell them!". Mathematics is an essential tool of science and each
scientific field develops mathematical tools adapted to its special needs.

REFERENCES

1. Thompson DW, On growth and form, Cambridge UP, London, 1961.

2. Sorenson J, Phelps M, Physics in Nuclear Medicine, Grune & Stratton, New York, London, Toronto, Sydney, San Francisco, 1980.

3. Diethelm L, Heuck F, Olsson O, Strnad F, Vieten H, Zuppinger A, Handbuch der Medizinischen Radiologie, Band XV, Teil 1A, Springer-Verlag, Berlin, Heidelberg, New York, 1980.

4. Rhodes B, Quality control in Nuclear Medicine, Mosby, St. Louis, 1977.

5. Boas M, Mathematical methods in the physical sciences, John Wiley & Sons, New York, London, Sydney, 1966.

MODEL STUDIES WITH DUAL LABELLING

G. LIMOURIS, M. MARINI

INTRODUCTION

The purpose of this study is to discuss the possible applications of a model involving dual isotope-studies of a ligand and in particular of Fluorescein. Selective accumulation of a radioactive substance within an organ is the main property upon which scintigraphic imaging is based. The possibility of a preferential localization may be the result of direct introduction of the isotope into the blood-stream supplying the organ or due to affinity of the ligand for a particular tissue. It is well known that there are six main biological mechanisms which are responsible for the localization of radiopharmaceuticals in various organs or physiological compartments. These are phagocytosis, cell sequestration, capillary blockade, simple or exchange diffusion, compartmental localization and active transport. Because our model is based upon the use of phosphorus-32 which localizes in tumours by active transport this biological mechanism has been specifically examined.

Active transport is the ability of a particular tissue to selectively concentrate a specific molecular species from the flux of materials passing through the tissue. In most instances, blood serves as the transport vehicle and it is the affinity of this particular organ for a certain type of reagent that produces the focal concentration known as active transport. The prime problem therefore is to find a carrier which will utilize one or more of the above mechanisms to localize in the target organ. Phosphorus-32, Iodine-123 en Fluorescein are theoretically chosen as the suitable radiopharmaceuticals and ligand respectively. This idea arose because it is well known that Phosphorus-32 uptake can be used as a measure of phosphate ion incorporation into DNA and RNA fractions in cell nuclei of newly formed nucleic acids (1). According to Homburger and Fishman (2) this metabolic function lies at the heart of malignant cell multiplication and therefore Phosphorus-32 uptake reflex the rate of malignant growth, a characteristic most unique amongst tracers for tumour localization.

Diiodofluorescein(^{131}I)

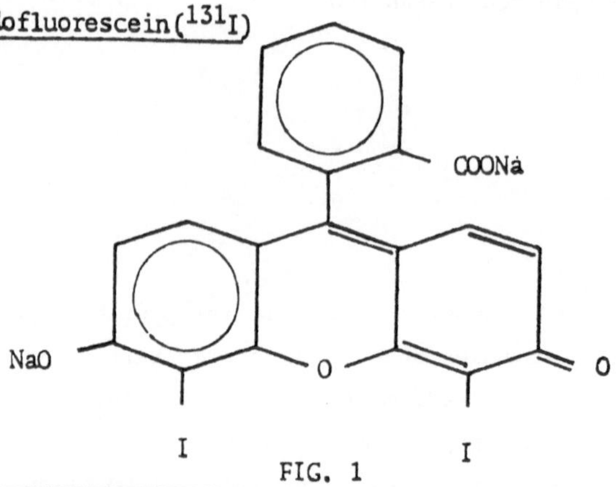

FIG. 1

Rose Bengal(^{131}I)

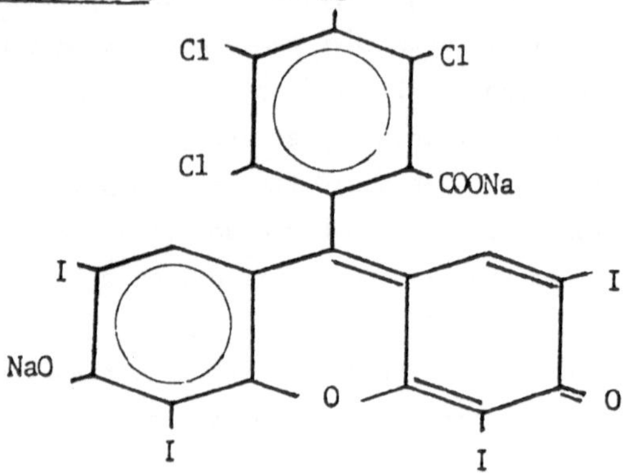

FIG. 2

Phosphate

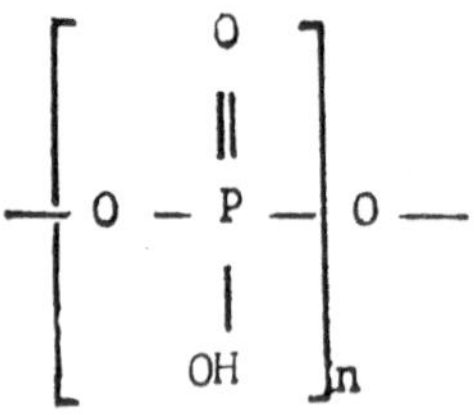

FIG. 3

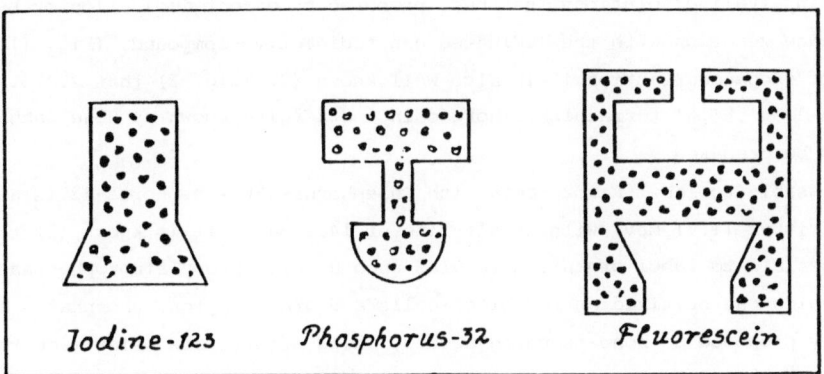

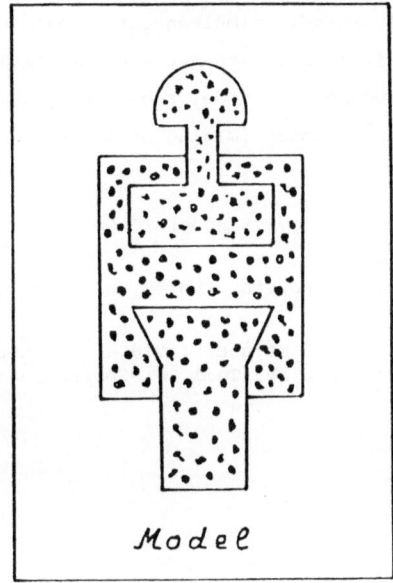

FIG. 4

From a pathophysiological point of view the tendency of the phosphate ion to concentrate to higher degree in malignant than in normal tissue and the tendency of normal tissues to clear Phosphorus-32 more rapidly than tumours explains its longer retention by tumours, a feature of great clinical importance. Les us now consider three aspects related to Fluorescein distribution:

- Is it possible to label Fluorescein with Iodine-123? It is know (1) that 4.5 Diiodofluorescein, a red-orange substance, insoluble in water in acid form soluble in alkaline solutions, has been prepared by direct iodination or by an exchange reaction with the iodinated non radioactive compound. (Fig. 1). By way of exchange reaction it is also well known (3) (fig. 2) that 2.4.5.7 tetraido-3',4',5',6' tetrachlorofluorescein - otherwise known as Rose Bengal can also be prepared.

- Is it possible to label Fluorescein with Phosphorus-32? Phosphorus-32 is a pure β-emitter (1.71 MeV) with a half-life of 14.3 days. It is known (3) tha it is possible to label organic molecules such as Diisopropylfluorophosphate (DFP), which can be fixed on red blood-cells and granulocytes. Phosphates ar currently proposed as bone scanning agents, while efforts are being made to extend them to biological tests. Experiences of the incorporation of Phos-phorus-32 into Fluorescein has not yet been reported (fig. 3).

- Is it possible to label Fluorescein simultaneously with two nuclides? In fig 4 one can see the fluorescein ligand with two nuclides bound to the proposed complex. The idea for producing this model substance arose because of techni problems involving the scintigraphic imaging of the eye.

REFERENCES

1. O'Rourke J, Nuclear Ophtalmology, Saunders Comp. Ltd. London, Philadelphia Toronto, 1976.

2. Homburger F, Fishman WH, The physiopathology of cancer, Hoeber Harper, New York, 1953, p. 584-585.

3. Diethelm L, Heuck F, Olsson O, Strnad F, Vieten H, Zuppinger A, Handbuch d Medizinischen Radiologie, Band XV, Teil 1A, Springer-Verlag, Berlin, Heide berg, New York, 1980.

AUTHOR INDEX

SUBJECT INDEX